Advance prais

T0352702

'Adolescence is a time of transition from chi_____ _____ during which there are rapid changes in physical, social, and emotional development. Coping with the onset of skin disease during this vulnerable time can be difficult. This is an excellent and much needed resource to support adolescents with skin disease by providing reliable information on common issues, addressing some of the myths around skin disease and promoting emotional wellbeing. An essential read for adolescents with skin disease and for the people who look after them.'
Dr Tanya Bleiker
President, British Association of Dermatologists (BAD), 2021

'The impact of skin diseases on people's lives can be profound due to their public visibility, commonly causing distress, anxiety, and embarrassment. Yet treatments mostly focus on the physical aspects, often neglecting the impact on our mental health. This is an excellent, much needed, and accessible book written with young people and the common skin problems they encounter in mind, easy to understand yet comprehensive and holistic in its approach.'
Professor Carsten Flohr
Chair in Dermatology & Population Health Sciences,
King's College London, UK
President, British Society for Paediatric Dermatology (BSPD), 2021

'A must-read for young people living with a skin condition and their families. This book provides clear and up-to-date information on a wide range of conditions while acknowledging their potential psychological and social impact on life. A highlight of the book, the final section, offers compassionate advice about living better, covering some crucial aspects of physical and mental health relevant to the reader. Each chapter shares a powerful message of hope and optimism, which young people struggling to cope with their skin condition desperately need.'
Magali Redding,
CEO, Eczema Outreach Support, UK

'*Skin conditions in young people* includes a fantastic guide to our skin condition, offering practical, achievable advice on managing your vitiligo and its impact on you. We were pleased to contribute to this book, which will help give young people the confidence to live comfortably in their vitiligo skin.'
Emma Rush,
CEO, Vitiligo Support, UK

'*Skin conditions in young people* embodies the values of both The Dipex Charity and healthtalk.org. By understanding a health condition holistically, both young patients and health professionals are better able to understand the wider impact of issues such as skin conditions and improve experiences and care.'
Adam Barnett,
CEO, The Dipex Charity, UK

Reader reviews

'I found it very useful, especially the final section about the mental side of skin conditions. I felt that I could relate to quite a few things in the book and it has helped me to cope with my scarring and speak to my parents more about the things I have been worrying about.'

Thomas, age 18 (acne)

'I found this so useful— it was information that had never been explained to me well. I am now managing my eczema so much better.'

Nadia, age 16 (eczema)

'I liked the simple message about eczema not being your fault, and that some-times it will flare for no reason. It's better not to drive yourself crazy trying to work out why it flared, but to just focus on getting on top of it and trying to not let it stop you doing the things you enjoy.'

Callum, age 13 (eczema)

'The HS chapter actually made me feel a bit better about the condition, especially in terms of feeling "dirty".'

Jessica, age 14 (hidradenitis suppurativa)

'Straight away I read the section "Living in your skin". This is something that I know I struggle with regardless of the fact that other people have far more severe psoriasis than me. Reading through it, I found that I have experienced so many of the feelings referenced. The typical "Why me" is a really common thought. Another is that I would feel happier without psoriasis. This is hard to deal with as it's very difficult to control. But knowing more ways to tackle these thoughts is useful. This was great to read and seemed to be really in line with feelings that I've experienced for a while.'

Luke, age 16 (psoriasis)

thefacts

Skin Conditions in Young People

➲ also available in thefacts series

the**facts**

Skin Conditions in Young People
A practical guide on how to be comfortable in your skin

Tess McPherson

Consultant Dermatologist, Oxford University Hospitals,
NHS Foundation Trust, Oxford, UK

Illustrations by
Damian Hale

Graphic Designer, London, UK

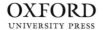
OXFORD
UNIVERSITY PRESS

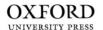

OXFORD
UNIVERSITY PRESS

Great Clarendon Street, Oxford, OX2 6DP,
United Kingdom

Oxford University Press is a department of the University of Oxford.
It furthers the University's objective of excellence in research, scholarship,
and education by publishing worldwide. Oxford is a registered trade mark of
Oxford University Press in the UK and in certain other countries

First Edition published in 2021

Impression: 1

Published in the United States of America by Oxford University Press
198 Madison Avenue, New York, NY 10016, United States of America

British Library Cataloguing in Publication Data
Data available

Library of Congress Control Number: 2021940636

ISBN 978–0–19–289542–4

DOI: 10.1093/oso/9780192895424.001.0001

Printed and bound by
CPI Group (UK) Ltd, Croydon, CR0 4YY

Acknowledgements

I would like to thank all who have offered their expertise in various chapters. I would like to give particular thanks to Su Bullus and Danny Simpson who reviewed and edited the whole book. Su is a very special, specialist nurse who has helped develop the services in Oxford for young people and is wise, sensible, and empathetic. Danny is now a junior doctor but I met as a student interested in paediatrics—I am not sure he realized the pamphlet I had in mind would turn into such a big project.

My family, especially the young people have been really helpful, and in particular Josie who helped edit chapters when she was stuck home in lockdown.

I am grateful to the many charities who have collaborated and advised on content including British Society of Paediatric Dermatology (BSPD), National Eczema Society (NES), Eczema Outreach Support (EOS), healthtalk.org (Dipex charity) and Vitiligo support. These provide support for dermatological conditions have been increasingly involved in specific needs of young people with skin conditions.

I am very fortunate to have been able to work with a psychologist and psychiatrist, Kate Chapman and Mina Fazel, respectively, who contributed to the section 'Living in your skin'. Kate and Mina have worked with me to develop services in Oxford to support managing young people's skin and impact on mental health. Kate and I run a monthly adolescent clinic which has shown that supporting psychological health alongside managing skin can lead to better outcomes for young people. Working with a psychologist has taught me the things that you don't always hear unless you ask the right questions, confirmed the need to support the psychological impact of skin conditions and really inspired the writing of this book.

Finally, I have learnt so much from the young people we work with in dermatology and the patients who shared their experiences in healthtalk.org; both their struggles and their amazing strength and resilience. Many have read sections of this book and advised and encouraged me to share these messages. Thank you all!

Contents

PART III
Living in your skin

Contributors

Susannah Baron
Consultant Dermatologist, Guy's
and St Thomas' NHS Foundation
Trust, UK
Chapter 16

Su Bullus
Specialist Paediatric Nurse, Oxford
University Hospitals, Oxford, UK
Chapters 1–17

Kate Chapman
Consultant Clinical Psychologist,
Oxford University Hospitals,
Oxford, UK
Chapters 15 and 16

Sharon Dixon
GP, Donnington Health Centre,
Oxford, UK
Chapter 5

Mina Fazel
Child and Adolescent Psychiatrist,
Oxford University, Oxford, UK
Chapters 15 and 16

Inge Kreuser-Genis
Consultant Dermatologist, Oxford
University Hospitals, Oxford, UK
Chapter 12

John Reed
Consultant Dermatologist, Oxford
University Hospitals, Oxford, UK
Chapter 5

Emma Rush
Vitiligo Support, UK
Chapter 11

Danny Simpson
Junior Doctor (Paediatrics),
Bristol, UK
Chapters 1–17

Part I

Introduction to skin

1

Introduction

Skin—it's amazing

It's a waterproof, breathable organ, made up of millions of cells that are all working hard to keep our body functioning. It covers us, holds us together, and protects us from the world.

Skin is also a window into our soul; our emotions are shown through it. We blush, we sweat, and we glow, especially when we're embarrassed or excited.

Beauty is not skin deep

We get judged on our skin, even though we know beauty is not just skin deep. The person we are doesn't depend on our skin; we should instead be judged on what lies beneath. That's what decides who we are, how we treat people, and how we treat ourselves.

How skin can cause problems

Skin can get itchy, scaly, dry, spotty, greasy, warty . . .

Developing a skin problem doesn't really have much to do with doing things wrong or not doing things right. We all inherit different skin, and so we each have a different chance of developing alopecia, psoriasis, or any other skin condition. It's a complex process, with many factors playing a role. Most conditions will therefore come and go throughout life, and this can be difficult to control.

The most important thing to remember is that it's not your fault. You shouldn't be wondering whether you've done something wrong, or if there was something you could have been doing differently. It's sometimes hard to deal with, it can be stressful, and it can really get you down.

Skin Conditions in Young People. Tess McPherson, Oxford University Press. © Oxford University Press 2021.
DOI: 10.1093/oso/9780192895424.003.0001

This book aims to help you with the things that **can** be done instead. It will teach you to take responsibility for yourself and your skin, how to cope when skin problems are difficult to manage, and how to deal with the stress that having a skin condition can bring. All of this should help you to get more comfortable in your skin (Fig. 1.1).

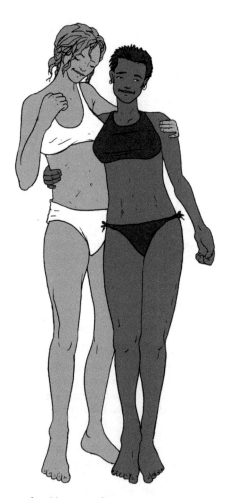

Figure 1.1 Feeling comfortable in your skin.
© Reproduced courtesy of Damian Hale.

2

Normal skin

 Key points

- Our skin is an amazing organ, and works pretty well most of the time.

- We all have different skin, and most of these differences are totally normal.

- We can all define what normal skin is; it doesn't have to be 'perfect' to be normal.

What is normal skin?

'Normal' skin (def): skin that works well, and that can do all the jobs that it needs to.

Skin is much more than just a wrapper that holds our bodies in place; it's a dynamic, active organ. Each of the organs in your body is made up of similar cells that work together, and in fact, your skin is the largest one of them all. The skin cells that it consists of are constantly on the go, and every month they are completely renewed.

Skin has so many roles to fulfil. It holds us together, acting as a responsive barrier that keeps the right things in and the wrong things out. It's home to a host of its own bugs, which work and live together, and it also does a pretty good job of fighting unwelcome infections. You have cells in your skin that will target problematic bugs, leaving just the friendlier ones behind.

Skin is a barrier to sunlight too, and can use the sun's rays to make the vitamin D we need to keep our bone strength up. Plus, if you're getting too much sun and start to feel a bit hot, your skin can fix that as well; by altering the amount of blood flowing to your skin you can either let heat out or keep it in. This is why your skin goes red when you're hot and white when you're cold.

Skin Conditions in Young People. Tess McPherson, Oxford University Press. © Oxford University Press 2021.
DOI: 10.1093/oso/9780192895424.003.0002

> **Box 2.1** Inflammation in the skin
>
> Inflammation is caused by increased activity of the immune cells in your body. These are the ones that hang around ready to fight infections and repair damage. They can become active even without an infection triggering things, which is often the problem in 'inflammatory' skin conditions. The process of inflammation causes increased blood flow, which means areas look redder or darker (this is called erythema although the colour will depend on skin pigment type), will be raised, and can be itchy or sore. It is important to understand that these **inflammatory conditions are not contagious or catching**—although you can pass on infections, you do **not pass on inflammation.**

Skin is pretty incredible, and thankfully just gets on with all these jobs most of the time. It can get damaged though, like any other organ, and become infected, inflamed (Box 2.1), or even cancerous. Many common skin conditions covered in this book can be managed with the right treatments. However, rarely skin really can't do its job—for example. after severe burn, or widespread skin disease. If skin stops working properly people can get really ill, and we're reminded how important normal, functioning, healthy skin can be.

The other reason that people worry so much about skin is that it is the bit of us that everyone can see, the face that we show to the world. This is where a different and more complicated kind of 'normal' comes in. What should normal skin look like? Who defines this anyway?

We all want to be 'normal'—this feels particularly important during teenage years, but to be honest, most adults think it too. You don't want to stand out in any way that is bad, and so that means being the same as everybody else. But do we all want to be the same? Normal skin includes many variants, and so even if we did all want identical skin it would be pretty much impossible. We are all different, inherit different genes, live in different environments, and all have different skin. Some differences are celebrated, some are not, but this varies across societies and changes massively over time. Beautiful skin in one part of the world might be totally ordinary somewhere else, and while admittedly there aren't many societies that celebrate spots or boils, even this could change. We—hopefully—now live in a time when people are more accepting of difference, and so there is no longer a clear definition of beauty or beautiful skin. There is certainly a reassuring trend emerging, and models and celebrities these days tend to be more varied in terms of looks; people who have no hair due to alopecia bare their scalps, for example, when some years ago this would have been considered unacceptable. Similarly, there is a black supermodel with a condition that causes skin to lose its colour (vitiligo), and her pigmentation changes are now seen as beautiful too.

However, if you've got vitiligo and you're not famous, the fact that there is now a celebrity who does have it might not make you feel that much better. Yes, some areas of the media celebrate conditions like these, but there are still lots of pictures and adverts, particularly on social media, that would suggest something totally different. They would have you believe that normal skin is flawless and glowing, that everybody should look perfect all of the time. And that's when your 'normal' skin starts to feel like it isn't good enough. If you're pale you should tan, if you're dark you should bleach. If you've got spots or a rash then these should definitely be covered up, or stop you doing things because nobody ever has those kinds of imperfections in the images we are exposed to.

Skin conditions like acne and eczema are rarely, if ever, seen in the media, so plenty of people think they're rare and abnormal. If you look at the numbers though, this is clearly a mistake. Over 90% of people get spots in adolescence, and about 1 in 5 have eczema at some point in their lives. Approximately 1 in 5 people are left-handed, but not many people think being left-handed is out of the ordinary; why should eczema be any different? When you look at these statistics, you have to ask what's really more common—the skin that you see on social media, or all the 'imperfect' skin you see in the real world around you?

Back to my definition of 'normal': *skin that works well, and that can do all the jobs it needs to.*

Normal skin is hairy and sweaty. Normal skin has freckles and moles on it, normal skin gets spots, normal skin gets rashes on it sometimes, and normal skin bears scars. We all have a say in what normal is, and normal cannot just be an unblemished, 'photoshopped' version of skin. Young people are in control of a lot of that, and will have a big part in deciding what kind of skin is judged to be normal and beautiful in the near future.

Skin doesn't have to look perfect in order to be healthy, and we certainly don't need to look the same in order to be beautiful. This book aims to help you look after your skin, with advice on how to manage some common conditions and help keep it functioning healthily. It is not here to make you think that the only way to be happy and healthy is to have skin with one pigment, no hair, no sweat, no moles, no freckles, no scars, and never any redness anywhere—that is **not** normal, and to be honest it's not even possible. If you're feeling bad about your skin, or other people are being negative about it, then we can definitely help. We won't, however, attempt to give you flawless skin, because that isn't normal; our differences are both interesting and necessary, and we shouldn't be trying to get rid of our variety.

Part II

Problem skin

3

Spots and acne

 Key points

- Getting spots is very common, and nearly all young people get spots to some degree.

- Spots in people with acne appear due to changes in something called the pilosebaceous gland, which becomes more active during puberty.

- There are lots of treatments available that can help to reduce spots.

What is acne?

Acne, a word that essentially means lots of spots, has been around for ages. Acne vulgaris is the term for 'common' acne which is the type most teenagers get. Acne rosacea is generally in slightly older adults and—as the name suggests—often involves redness of the skin alongside the spots. The word acne is actually a mistranslation of the Greek word *acme*, which means 'peak' or high point. This refers to the peaks of the spots—not that having acne is a high point for many people.

You do not get spots because you are dirty and eat junk. Spots appear due to hormonal changes which effect the skin. These happens to everybody going through puberty, so everyone gets spots; even if it feels like other people have perfect skin most of the time (Fig. 3.1).

Introduction to the pilosebaceous unit

Humans are mammals, and one feature that most mammals share is that—apart from our palms and soles—our skin is covered with hairs. Each skin pore or hair follicle contains a hair and a tiny gland, which releases sweat along with a greasy substance called sebum. The hair follicles are useful in keeping us at the right temperature, and the sebum helps keep skin moisturized and working

Skin Conditions in Young People. Tess McPherson, Oxford University Press. © Oxford University Press 2021.
DOI: 10.1093/oso/9780192895424.003.0003

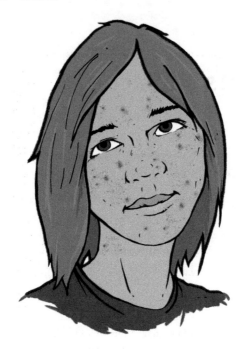

Figure 3.1 Spots.
© Reproduced courtesy of Damian Hale.

effectively as a barrier. Extra sebum production though, which often happens in puberty, can make skin greasy and more spot prone.

Together, the hair in the follicle and the gland that produces sebum are called the pilosebaceous unit (Fig. 3.2) and any of these pilosebaceous units can form a spot. We have more of these 'units' and they are more active on the face—particularly the forehead, nose, and chin—the chest and the back, and this is why we tend to get more spots in these areas. Hormones influence the production of sebum by the sebaceous gland. More sebum means clogging of the pores and this is when spots can develop. Other factors play a role including a particular skin bug known as *Cutibacterium acnes (C. acnes)*; which seems to like sebum-rich skin.

Why me?

There is no simple answer as to why some people are more prone to spots than others. It's all down to the differences in the activity of your pilosebaceous

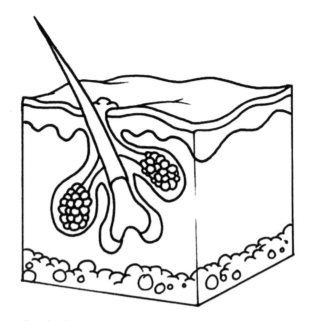

Figure 3.2 The pilosebaceous unit—each skin pore has a hair and a sebaceous gland which makes up a potential spot forming unit.
© Reproduced courtesy of Damian Hale.

units. This is the result of many things, including what your parents' skin is like, the skin you were born with, the hormones in your body, and the environment you live in. More 'developed' countries have higher rates of spots and it's not really clear why—it might have something to do with differences in diet. However, one thing is certain, and that is that almost every teenager in the UK gets spots to some degree.

Clean skin and spots

Washing your face is important, and can help reduce grime and grease to some extent. Spots are not due to dirty skin, however, and people who wash regularly can still get severe acne.

Diet and spots

A healthy diet is good for us for many reasons, but that doesn't mean that junk food is the cause of acne. Having said this, high levels of certain food types can be linked to spots; a diet that is low in fat and sugar—known as a 'low gly-caemic diet'—can reduce acne in some people, and there is now good evidence that consumption of high amounts of dairy can make some people more spot prone. This isn't the only reason that people are more likely to get spots, how-ever, and reducing dairy may or may not help your skin. Remember, vegans can get acne too!

Hormones

Hormones are substances that are produced naturally in our bodies, and have plenty of important roles. The most important of all these hormones in acne are called the 'sex hormones'; these are the ones that change a lot around puberty.

A group of sex hormones known as androgens are particularly involved. You might have heard of testosterone, which is just one example of an androgen, but there are also loads of other androgens—not just testosterone—that help to control things like bone strength, muscle growth, and emotional well-being.

They are present in both males and females, although usually at higher levels in males, and the levels increase during puberty. It's this increase, which is generally bigger in boys, that causes more sebum to be produced by that pilosebaceous unit; frustratingly, it makes you more spot prone just as you are dealing with all the other bits of development too.

Female hormone changes, relating to the menstrual cycle and pregnancy, can also have an effect on acne. There are certain patterns of acne—especially spots along the jawline—that can be particularly bad around your period.

As these hormone changes during puberty are different for boys and girls, the skin changes that we usually see are different too. Boys have a higher chance of bad acne, and this more commonly resolves by the end of puberty; girls are less commonly affected by severe acne meanwhile, but do have a higher risk of more persistent acne. It can last until—or even start in—their twenties and thirties.

Other important hormones and acne

Polycystic ovary syndrome (PCOS)

This is a hormonal abnormality seen in some women, and it can be anything from mild to really severe. Higher than normal androgen levels are found in women with this condition, which can lead to irregular periods, weight gain, extra hair growth, and a higher chance of acne.

Anabolic steroid supplements

Anabolic steroids are synthetic hormones, not naturally made in the body, that have the same effect as natural testosterones. They can be bought quite easily over the internet, and are being used by young people more often nowadays to help promote muscle growth. They can increase acne. They also come with many other potential health risks, so these should not be used without correct supervision. Do tell your doctor if you are using supplements; they will not judge you, but it will affect how they treat your skin.

Transgender skin

If you are prescribed hormones for gender transition, these can affect your skin. Taking the male hormones can make you more spot prone—as well as having the desired effects of transition—which is something that you might want to discuss treatment for with your doctor.

Stress hormones

It may seem like you get more spots when you are stressed. There is evidence that this could be the case for some people, as a hormone called cortisol, released when we're stressed, can act in a similar way to androgens and trigger outbreaks in those prone to acne.

What is certainly true is that having an outbreak—particularly when you have a big event on—can make you even more stressed. Then, because you're not feeling great, you might focus on your skin and spots and start a vicious cycle. Having said that, a little bit of stress isn't necessarily a bad thing and so it may not be that simple; plus, some stressed people seem to get no spots at all. It's all a bit complicated, but given that there might be a link there, managing your skin and helping with how you feel in yourself can, and should, be addressed at the same time (Chapter 17).

Types of spots involved in acne

Spots can come in many different forms (Fig. 3.3), and you could have mostly one type or a mixture of them all. It's also important to remember that some of these types can cause scars, so treatment should be considered to both prevent spots and to avoid scarring.

Comedones

You might sometimes see whiteheads and blackheads referred to as comedones (Figs. 3.3a and b). These are often the first spots you get, but can be seen in all stages of mild, moderate, or severe acne.

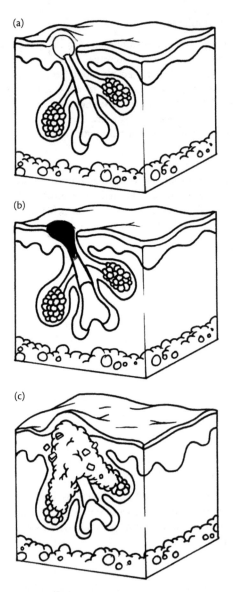

(a)

(b)

(c)

Figure 3.3 Different types of spots: (a) whitehead (closed comedone); (b) blackhead (open comedone); and (c) pustule.

© Reproduced courtesy of Damian Hale.

Comedones form when the hair follicle gets full of gunk, which tends to be mostly sebum. Closed comedones are known as whiteheads, whereas blackheads are called open comedones, because in this case the pore becomes open to the air. This causes the sebum—which is white normally—to turn black when exposed to oxygen, and so this explains why whiteheads and blackheads look the way they do.

Papules, pustules, cysts, and nodules

Papules, pustules, cysts, and nodules (Fig. 3.3c) are all types of 'inflammatory lesions'. This is just another way of saying that the immune cells in your body—the ones that fight infections and repair damage—are hanging around in the skin, causing more blood flow (erythema), swelling, and pus (Box 2.1). The bacteria *C. acnes;* which thrives in the greasy conditions provided by sebum, might also be present; this then brings even more of the immune cells to the area and worsens the problem.

Papules are little red bumps that can settle on their own, whereas pustules are the squeezable, pus-filled ones (should you squeeze or not?—see Box 3.1). Pus is thicker than sebum and contains a particular form of immune cell, a white blood cell called a neutrophil.

Cysts and nodules are bigger spots, which can be painful and deep under the skin. These are seen in more severe acne, and may mean that tablet treatments should be considered.

Box 3.1 Squeezing and picking

OK—so if you have one big pustule, then it is probably OK to squeeze it. Clean your hands first, and wash your face after. There are whole websites devoted to squeezing spots, and clearly some people love doing this, but maybe don't try and make it a regular hobby.

What is not so helpful is picking at small spots, and trying to get rid of every little spot before it's inflamed. This will probably make them more inflamed if anything—rather than help them heal—and could also make marks and scars more likely. Spots can scar even if you don't touch them though, so if you're concerned that spots are causing scars then this is a reason to see your doctor.

Post-inflammatory marks

The 'inflammatory lesions' mentioned earlier often leave marks. Recently healed spots can lead to flat, redder marks that will fade, and any lighter or darker patches of skin that appear after a spot will also usually fade over time.

Spots can also leave scars, which could either be raised on top of the skin or sunken into it. Picking and squeezing can make scars more likely, but even if you don't squeeze your spots they can still cause scarring. This is one of the important reasons to treat severe acne, because this is when scarring most often occurs. Thankfully the majority of scars will improve over time, but the best thing is to try and reduce acne activity, to prevent them from forming in the first place.

How to manage spots and acne

Some people are OK with getting the odd spot, or even with getting quite a few; that is absolutely fine. It is, after all, a completely normal part of growing up.

It's fine to wear make-up, and some products can be helpful in covering up spots to make you feel better. It's sensible to wash off make-up at the end of the day though, and you should try and find a make-up that works for your skin; products that are labelled 'non-comedogenic' have less oil, do not occlude hair pores so much, and therefore better for spot prone skin.

If your skin is becoming problematic, however—for example, because you've got lots of spots, constant spots, painful spots, spots leaving scars, or any kind of spots that are stopping you feeling OK about doing the things that you normally would want to—then you should think about what you can do to help.

What you can do

If your spots aren't too bad then they are likely to improve over time. Keeping skin clean is important, as is trying not to squeeze or pick spots if you can avoid it.

A healthy diet, with enough fruit and vegetables, will probably benefit your health, and—as mentioned before—certain people might benefit from cutting down on high-sugar and dairy products if they're consuming a lot of those.

If your spots are severe or affecting you too much though, then this might be the time to start thinking about other treatments that are available. You have plenty of options, which you can get over the counter at a pharmacy, online, or on prescription from your GP or dermatologist. There are two main types of treatment that we use: either topical creams and ointments, or tablets.

Topical treatments

Several topical treatments have been shown to help spots; you have lots to choose from, but remember that, because everyone's skin is different, you may not like what other people recommend. Buying expensive stuff is not necessarily better; despite what they say, there may only be limited evidence for a lot of the claims that these products make on the packaging.

Topical treatments generally work by stopping new spots, so need to be applied to all spot-prone skin in order to prevent new ones from forming. For this reason, they can take a bit of time to work, and it may feel like your skin is getting worse rather than better to start with. The creams and ointments aim to reduce how greasy your skin is, so are likely to make your skin dry and irritated—particularly when you first start using them. This should settle with continued use, but you may want to build up contact time slowly by using them just a few nights a week to start with.

There are a few medications that work in this way, and they are all described next. Each contains a different 'active ingredient', which you can check for on the back of the packet before you buy. Most of these are prescription products available from a doctor, but some are available over the counter. Many are also now available online. These online versions may have lower concentrations of the active ingredients however, so you should always be careful where you are buying things from. Find a reliable supplier, with products that actually contain what they claim to!

Benzoyl peroxide

Effective at preventing and treating spots. It has been around for ages, and is therefore cheap. Potential downsides are that it can cause irritation initially, plus it bleaches things; you therefore need to be careful with pillows and towels. It's available over the counter in the UK.

Topical retinoids

These are effective for all types of spots. If you've only got comedones, retinoids are the best treatment to go for as they can also make your pores tighter. They usually need to be on prescription, but certain variants are available online. These should be avoided if you are pregnant or considering getting pregnant but can otherwise be used for years if necessary, and can be very effective in preventing spots.

Topical antibiotics

These help with inflammatory acne; the papules, pustules, cysts, and nodules. They work by reducing the number of those immune cells hanging around in the skin, and also by targeting the *C. acnes* bacteria that causes more of these cells to appear. Bugs like *C. acnes* can become resistant to this kind of treatment, so longer use of topical or tablet antibiotics is not recommended. Topical antibiotics are best used for short courses and alongside retinoids, either as creams or tablets, to help prevent this.

Combination treatments

If you have more than one type of spot, as people commonly do, then a combined treatment is usually best. These are normally available on prescription from your GP; they might give you gels or creams containing both a topical retinoid and benzoyl peroxide, for example, or both a topical retinoid and an antibiotic.

Oral treatments

If spots are bad, not controlled with topical treatments, or affecting areas that are hard to apply topical treatment to—such as your back or chest—then tablets should probably be considered. Again, as with the topical treatments, there are a few different options available.

Oral antibiotics

These can be helpful for acne that is inflamed or widespread. Just like the topical antibiotics, they work by reducing inflammation, as well targeting the bugs that play a role in this. A course of these antibiotics will be longer than you would normally take for a throat or chest infection; it will probably last 3–6 months, and you'll most likely be given antibiotics called either lymecycline or oxytetracycline. As with the topical antibiotics, your course should not be any longer than this. Resistance of bacteria can develop, meaning the antibiotics won't work as well for you, or for other people with serious infections. Antibiotic resistance is a major global problem, and we need to use antibiotics sensibly.

Some people respond excellently to a course of antibiotics, and their spots will often improve. If this is the case for you, it will hopefully be enough to take you through your spot-prone period. Other people don't get much benefit however, or have acne that quickly comes back when the course is finished; in these situations, it might be time to try a different type of treatment.

Oral contraceptive pill and spironolactone

Sometimes hormonal treatment can be useful in females, in particular if spots seem to flare with period cycle. The combined contraceptive pill can be used alongside oral antibiotic or oral retinoid tablets. Spironolactone—sometimes just called 'spiro'—is a tablet that has an antiandrogen effect, and can be helpful in female patients with hormonal acne that continues after puberty.

Oral retinoids

If acne is severe, not improving, and showing signs of scarring, or if it involves deeper cysts or nodules, there is a treatment available known as isotretinoin *(often called Roaccutane, which is the original brand name of the drug)* that can be very effective. This is currently only available through the hospital dermatologist. Isotretinoin is a retinoid, which is essentially a tablet made from vitamin A; this is the same vitamin you get from carrots, but you would have to eat hundreds of carrots to get the same dose.

Not everyone with spots needs the oral retinoid tablet. Most people don't, and can be managed by topical treatments, oral antibiotics, or the contraceptive pill and time.

Although it's not really a 'stronger' tablet, it is the most effective treatment for acne. The reason it's only available in hospitals is that it's a relatively new treatment, although having said this, it has been in use for almost 30 years. Your mum or dad may even have taken it when they were your age. Over this fairly short time it has been mainly specialists who have become familiar with the medication, and so they are the ones responsible for prescribing it.

Isotretinoin reduces sebum, and minimizes the 'clogging' of your hair follicles. The dose you are prescribed will depend on a variety of factors; how bad your acne is, whether you have a tendency to develop dry skin or eczema, and how much you weigh, for example. A higher dose taken for a shorter time may cause more side effects, but you could get through the treatment quicker. Lower doses are likely to cause less problems with dry skin on the other hand, but you may end up taking tablets for longer. It works well in a lot of cases, and the majority of people will stop getting new spots over a 4–6 month course. The good part is that for most—around 6 to 7 out of 10—this is a sustained response; they remain less spot prone going forward, and some never get acne again.

So, is there a catch?

In general, isotretinoin is well tolerated and most people do fine with it. A lot of the common side effects are related to the dose you take, which will depend on your weight and diet. The dose can be adjusted depending on how bad the spots are, how dry and sensitive your skin is, and how much the medication is helping.

Common and important side effects of isotretinoin

Skin side effects

Isotretinoin can commonly make spots flare up a bit at the beginning. This generally only lasts a week or two, and can be improved by starting on lower doses initially. In addition, the treatment makes you more sensitive to sunburn; be careful if on holiday, and especially at festivals, as you end up being outside for long periods of time with no shade.

Isotretinoin also causes dry skin to some degree, as this is how it works. Thankfully this can usually be managed with moisturizers, but if it's severe the dose can be reduced. This might be a little bit annoying, but if your spots are bad it can be easier to take a tablet like this to help stop new spots, and then use moisturizers to treat dryness. The alternative is having to use two or three different creams to do different things on your skin, which can be more of a pain to deal with.

Pregnancy-related side effects

Isotretinoin can cause severe problems to developing babies. You must not get pregnant while taking this tablet. This will be discussed with you by the hospital dermatologist if you are going to be prescribed isotretinoin, and is one of the reasons that you should be under specialist care.

Tattoos, piercings, and hair removal

Because your skin becomes a bit dry on this treatment, it can be more easily irritated; stuff like laser hair removal, tattoos, and piercings should therefore probably be avoided. You can wax or shave your hair with appropriate moisturizer use, but it might depend on what dose you are on and how dry your skin gets. Remember you can always discuss this with your doctor if you're worried.

Blood results

You will probably be asked to get some blood tests to check on your liver, and to measure the fat levels in your blood. These should be normal before starting the tablet. They will be checked again after a month or two on the treatment, and if they're normal at this point you usually won't need more tests.

We test your liver function because the tablet is passed through your liver, as are many other medications. Alcohol is a toxin which is also cleared through the liver, so it is recommended that you avoid 'heavy' drinking while you're on this treatment; this is to make sure your liver isn't being put under too much strain.

A short course of isotretinoin will not cause problems in the majority, especially as young people are usually healthy. It's not yet known whether longer courses of this tablet could have an impact on fat levels in the blood further down the line, and so this is an area currently being researched; otherwise, the treatment appears to work well for most. If you have other health issues, or are on other medications however, this will need to be discussed with your doctor before you start taking isotretinoin.

Does isotretinoin cause mental health issues?

This has been a long-running debate, and the answer is still not completely clear.

When this tablet was first used, there were possible links made to severe depression and even suicide. It should be pointed out however, that the tablet—like a lot of new medications—was originally only used in people with very severe acne, and generally at higher doses than we use today.

In the 30 years since, these possible links have been well studied; it is now clear that this is not an expected side effect, and most people have no problems when on the medication. Comparing groups of young people who have taken the tablet with those who have not, there are similar rates of low mood in both. We know that this age is a vulnerable time, and low mood, anxiety, and depression are common. We also know that having skin problems can have a major influence on your mood, and that's one of the reasons this book was written in the first place. Some recent studies actually show that young people with severe acne are more likely to feel better in themselves if their skin has improved—which makes sense—following treatment with isotretinoin.

Mood changes may occur in certain individuals, as a rare and very occasional side effect. This is unpredictable, so if you feel in any way different or unwell then you should always tell someone; you could also contact your doctor if you have any concerns. This is true of nearly every medication, and is one of the reasons that if you don't need tablets it is best not to take them. If you are likely to benefit however, then you probably should. Remember that with any tablets you have to consider the benefits versus the risks, so have a look at the information available online and discuss this with your doctor. This should help you to work out whether the treatment is right for you.

Scars

Scars can only be treated when your acne is no longer active. The first and most important thing is to get treatment that will stop new spots; when you are no longer getting new spots, any marks or scars can then be assessed. Treatments to stop spots will not change existing scars, but should help prevent any further scarring.

Time may be the best treatment for some marks. Your body, and in particular your skin, is pretty amazing at healing itself. Simple skin care with appropriate moisturizers can help this process, but if you have very bumpy or pitted scars then there are treatments that could be discussed. These treatments are not available on the NHS, but your doctor or dermatologist can still point you in the right direction.

Resources

Young people's experiences of acne:

http://healthtalk.org/young-peoples-experiences/acne/topics

Acne support website set up by the British Association of Dermatologists:

http://www.acnesupport.org.uk/

Information on isotretinoin:

https://www.bad.org.uk/patient-information-leaflets/isotretinoin

4

Dry skin and eczema

 Key points

- People have different degrees of 'dryness' to their skin.

- Some inherited conditions, such as ichthyosis, can cause skin to be prone to becoming dry.

- Eczema is characterized by skin that is dry and easily inflamed.

- Atopic eczema is the most common type of eczema, and affects up to 1 in 5 people.

- People with atopic eczema can have a lifelong risk of sensitive skin that is also prone to flare-ups.

- Allergy testing is only required in certain cases; it will not change the type of skin you have, or the fact that your eczema needs treating.

- There are plenty of evidence-based treatments available that can help control and manage eczema.

Dry skin

We all have different skin. Some people might have skin that's a bit greasier, for example, or others may have skin that tends to be dry. Skin becomes 'dry' when it struggles to act as a good barrier, meaning all the moisture normally held by the skin is lost. This could be simply because a person has inherited a tendency to dry skin from their parents, or their skin might instead have been exposed to things in the environment that cause dryness. Whatever the cause, emollients or moisturizers can be used to help reduce dryness (see later), and are likely to have to be used regularly.

Skin Conditions in Young People. Tess McPherson, Oxford University Press. © Oxford University Press 2021.
DOI: 10.1093/oso/9780192895424.003.0004

Keratosis pilaris

Keratosis pilaris (KP) is the medical name for an extremely common form of dry, bumpy skin, which causes the hair follicles to become a bit dry and scaly. Sometimes called 'chicken skin' or goosebumps, it's really a variation on normal; it affects around 40% of adults and as many as 75% of young people, and is a result of inherited differences that often runs in families.

KP tends to affect the tops of the arms and legs, but can also be seen less commonly on the face and elsewhere. It doesn't generally cause any itch and is not a harmful condition, although KP can sometimes be seen with other dry skin conditions like ichthyosis or eczema.

If you think treatment might be needed, emollient creams that contain substances including salicylic acid, lactic acid, and/or urea are more effective in reducing dryness and scale than standard emollients, and can be either bought over the counter or prescribed by the doctor. Gentle exfoliation might be helpful in making skin feel less dry and rough too.

What is ichthyosis?

Ichthyoses are inherited conditions that leads to skin dryness. Some affect just the skin, whereas others might be associated with further differences in hair and teeth, for example. Ichthyosis develops as a result of inherited alterations in the skin, which lead to lifelong dry skin that requires lots of regular moisturizing. The most common form is called ichthyosis vulgaris (IV), and people with this type may be at increased risk of KP and eczema too.

What is eczema?

Eczema in Greek means 'boiling over', which sums it up pretty well—it's that dry, inflamed, often itchy skin, and most people will get it at some point in their lives. There are a fair few different types (all with similar names), so it can get a bit confusing. To make matters worse we often use the word 'dermatitis' to refer to eczema, but they mean exactly the same thing.

Listed next are the different types of eczema that commonly affect young people; some categories overlap, and so the treatments can be very similar.

- *Atopic eczema (or atopic dermatitis)*—this is the most common form of eczema and will be what most of the section focuses on. It is often just called eczema.

◆ *Discoid eczema*—a form of eczema where, rather than symmetrical areas of inflamed skin on both sides of your body, you can get random small patches of skin affected. Certain bacteria can sometimes be a particular problem in discoid eczema, and treatments may need to target this.

◆ *Seborrheic eczema*—eczema which affects the 'seborrheic' areas. These areas have lots of the glands that produce natural oil to cover your skin; they are also the same places that are prone to spots and acne. Certain yeasts that live on the skin thrive in these areas, and treatment may include targeting them.

◆ *Contact eczema*—eczema which has developed because skin has reacted to something it has come into contact with. Irritant contact eczema is due to things that irritate the skin like soap or alcohol gel and we are all prone to. Allergic contact dermatitis is due to a specific 'allergic' reaction to a substance and is less common.

There are a few other types of eczema, including asteatotic (dry) eczema and venous eczema, but these are more common in older people.

What is atopic eczema/dermatitis?

Atopic dermatitis, often just called 'eczema', is a common inflammatory skin condition (Box 2.1). If you have eczema, or are prone to eczema, you have skin that tends to be dry and can get 'flare-ups'. These are when the skin gets inflamed; becomes redder or darker than normal skin and itchy. The areas that are most commonly affected by flare-ups are the creases of the arms and legs ('flexures') (Fig. 4.1) and the face, but if it's really bad then it can appear all over the body.

People sometimes expect children to 'grow out' of eczema, so it can feel very disappointing to still have eczema in your teens and adulthood. Not many young people ever get a good explanation of what eczema is, or how best to manage it—it may just have been explained to their parents when they were younger, or it may never have been explained very well at all. People sometimes feel they are given pots and tubes of different creams and have little idea why they are doing it. Many people think they have done or are doing things wrong to have eczema. As is the case for a lot of skin conditions, there is plenty of false information often passed around; hopefully this section will clear up the things that often cause confusion, and provide advice for looking after your skin that is based on good evidence instead.

The more we know about eczema the more complicated it seems to be and is certainly a complex and variable condition. However, there are a few facts

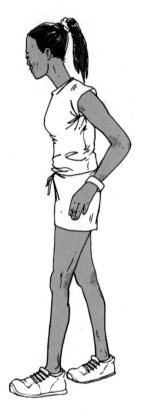

Figure 4.1 Eczema often flares in the creases of the arms and legs—'flexures'.
© Reproduced courtesy of Damian Hale.

which I find can help people understand eczema and mean they manage their skin better.

Eczema is caused by a complicated mix of inherited and environmental factors that affect the barrier function of the skin (skin is more 'leaky') and the way the immune system works (cells that cause inflammation are overactive and can overrespond to things in the environment and infections).

There is no 'cure' for eczema—this means you generally can't change the fact that you are prone to eczema. Because skin is leakier and the immune system is more active, eczema skin is prone to:

- Getting dry;
- Getting inflamed (flare-ups) often with no clear trigger.

Eczema can be associated with other 'atopic' conditions like hay fever, asthma, and food allergies. We call these conditions **atopic** and atopy is something that runs in families. These conditions occur because skin is leaky so can be easier for things in the environment to get exposed to the immune system and the immune system can overreact to these things. However, getting allergy tests is not needed for most people with eczema and generally will not change the fact that you have to manage eczema to some degree (see later).

Why haven't I grown out of eczema?

You may wonder why you?

You were probably told you would 'grow out of it'.

It is really important to know that you are not responsible for having eczema. It is not anything you have (or haven't done). We know eczema starts early in life and the reasons for this are complex. There are several known alterations to important genes which influence this and a load of possible environmental triggers. What's pretty clear is that although some people find their eczema improves, most people do not truly ever 'grow out' of eczema. Even if you have had years with just a bit of dry skin or no real problems with your skin it may get worse or flare-up—often for not clear reason. Annoyingly it seems to affect the face in adolescence. This persistence and uncertainty of eczema can be very frustrating: as one young person says:

'It's like the bad guy in a movie who just doesn't die.'

It is important to remember:

Just because there is no 'cure' does not mean it cannot be controlled.

Just because you are prone to eczema does not mean it cannot be managed.

Why can't I have tests to find the cause of my eczema?

We get asked this all the time and it is a bit complicated. As explained, people with eczema do have differences to the way their skin and immune system works. They are more likely to have asthma, hay fever, and sometimes food allergies. People frequently feel that if only they could find out what they were 'allergic' to, they would be able to sort their eczema. It certainly would be great if a simple allergy test could find one 'cause'—you could identify it, avoid it, and have no more issues. Unfortunately, it is rarely that simple. Eczema is, as we mentioned, a very complex condition, and most of the time there is no one

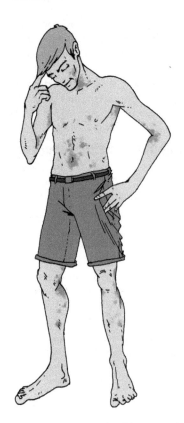

Figure 4.2 Atopic eczema—most young people with eczema do not need allergy tests.
© Reproduced courtesy of Damian Hale.

identifiable trigger. Allergy testing is only useful in specific circumstances, and generally does not change the fact your skin is prone to eczema (Fig. 4.2). This can be quite complicated, however, and sometimes causes a lot of confusion, so we will try and explain as best we can.

Food allergy and eczema (see hives and urticaria)

If you are truly allergic to a food, then eating it will cause an immediate reaction. You might have to avoid nuts, for example, because they cause a sudden rash—worse even, they could cause swelling of your lips, eyes, and problems with your breathing (Chapter 5). We now know that the majority of food al-lergies develop after eczema, rather than causing eczema to appear and are likely to be identified in childhood, and are much less likely to start in your teenage years.

Certain foods can make eczema worse for some people, but they generally take a bit of time to cause a problem; it's a matter of hours to days, rather than an instant change. There is no blood test for these types of reactions, and tests that may be offered (hair tests for example) are not reliable. If you really feel that a food (for example, dairy) seems to make your skin worse, then it may be worth a trial of exclusion to see if your skin does actually improve. We wouldn't recommend restricting your diet unnecessarily, and if you are going to try re-moving foods then you should do this one food at a time, avoiding each food for at least 4–6 weeks. You may have already tried this when you were younger and if it didn't change things much this is unlikely to be very useful.

Airborne allergies

Having atopy and atopic eczema does mean that you are likely to 'overreact' to harmless things in the environment, like dust, animal hair, and pollens—allergy tests for these would likely be positive in many people with eczema. You may already know that you get hay fever or asthma, and that this can be worse at certain times of year. You may also recognize that being with hairy pets or in a dusty place makes you sneeze, and even causes your eczema to get worse. It's important to understand however, that these reactions have not caused the eczema. Our understanding is that you are prone to these reactions because you are atopic and have eczema, not the other way around. Allergy testing will not be very useful, because even if it is positive, and even if reacting to these things may play a role in triggering your eczema, they are generally impossible to avoid completely. You can try steering clear of things if possible; getting rid of your hairy dog might not improve things much, but it's probably best not to go out and get a new one. You can't live in a world without trees, grass, and dust though, so you are going to have to live with them—the best strategy is therefore to manage the eczema with appropriate treatments.

Contact eczema—reacting to things on skin

Irritant contact eczema

Some creams can irritate your skin, spot treatments in particular—this is actu-ally how they're designed to work. If you have dry, sensitive skin then this type of irritant reaction can be more common, and could be triggered by anything from soap to tomatoes. The reaction happens quite quickly after your skin is exposed and can be worse during a flare-up when skin is already inflamed. This is often quite a helpful clue; it indicates that this is not an allergic reaction, and probably does not need allergy testing.

Allergic contact eczema

Other substances can cause a different type of skin reaction called allergic contact eczema, also known as contact dermatitis. In this case it's not soaps or tomatoes that's usually to blame—instead things like nickel (in cheap metal jewellery), fragrances, hair dye, nail varnishes are more often the cause. It's no more common in people with atopic eczema, and can happen to anyone; however, it does look very similar to atopic eczema, and so it can be hard to tell the difference sometimes. It only occurs in parts of your skin that have been in contact with the substance you're allergic too though, and so there are patterns that can give us clues—nail varnishes can affect the eyelids and neck, for example, as that is where you often touch your skin.

Unlike in irritant contact eczema, the reaction takes a few days to develop in most cases. If you suspect it is more likely to be an allergic reaction then you should be seen by your doctor, and a form of allergy testing called 'patch testing' will probably be organized. This involves putting small amounts of all the possible causes onto the skin on your back, and then reviewing the skin's response. It has to happen over a week, because—as we mentioned—the skin can take a few days to recognize the substance and cause a reaction.

You should also be aware that creams labelled 'organic' or 'natural' may well contain things that can cause an allergic contact eczema. Research has shown that these products are actually more likely to contain known allergens, like fragrances and preservatives, and are at risk of making your skin worse rather than better.

What causes flare-ups?

Flare-ups of eczema can make skin feel very itchy and have a massive effect on sleeping and how you feel. The uncertainty of when skin is going to flare-up can feel very frustrating. Understandably people try and work out what they can avoid to prevent them happening. Eczema-prone skin will overreact to a wide variety of things that normally wouldn't affect other people so much; pollen, soaps, bugs in skin, stress (Chapter 17)—there's a very long list of things thought to cause eczema to flare. If you have found things that seem to be responsible for flares and you can easily avoid them, that's great, but it isn't the case for most people. In fact, mostly **flare-ups just reflect the fact that eczema skin is easily inflamed and can be for no obvious reason at all.** Understanding this can actually be quite liberating. It means you can stop wondering what has flared your skin (may not be a simple answer or any answer) and instead focus on how to manage the skin (generally achievable) and get on with what you enjoy doing.

Don't worry: Dry skin and eczema can be managed.

Although eczema is a chronic, complex condition which sounds quite scary. Fortunately, the management can be pretty simple. This is achieved by

1. Targeting dryness
2. Treating the inflammation

Most people can do this with topical treatments (which are applied to the skin), but occasionally if this cannot control the eczema then there may be a need for tablets or injections.

Manage dryness (for eczema and all dry skin types)

Avoid irritants and use emollients

Many things irritate the skin even in people who don't have eczema. Eczema skin is particularly 'sensitive' and you probably will find that some products that other people can use may not suit your skin. This may include cleaning products, cosmetic products, and synthetic clothing. These products can irritate people even if they don't have 'sensitive' skin. If your skin is already prone to dryness though, this reaction is likely to be worse. This doesn't have to be complete avoidance but being a bit careful in particular if your skin is active. Anything which bubbles—soap, shower gel, fragrances—might make eczema worse, and so using an emollient when you wash can help prevent dryness.

Emollients (or moisturizers) (Box 4.1) help the skin to act as a barrier, which we know it has trouble doing in people with eczema and other drying skin conditions. They should be used regularly, but exactly how often is different for different people. Using enough to keep the skin from getting dry is the main thing. There are a whole range of emollients to choose from, but generally the less ingredients and fragrances the better. It's also important to be aware that just because a moisturizer is 'natural' and organic, it does not make it any better for eczema.

Emollients can feel like a pain to apply when you are busy. We find that doing it just once or twice a day, and even simply using one instead of soap to wash, can

---

Box 4.1 Guide to emollients

- Lotions: thin and easy to spread, but the least moisturizing.

- Creams (water-based): not very greasy and quickly absorbed, slightly more moisturizing.

- Ointments (oil-based): very thick and greasy, but also very moisturizing— need to be careful not to use them on very damaged areas though.

- Soap substitutes: many emollients can be used to wash your hands, or in the shower or bath. They don't make a foam like normal soap, but clean just as effectively.

---

be enough for some people. There is no evidence that applying emollient six, seven, or even more, times per day is needed, and this can actually cause problems rather than solve them—especially if no appropriate anti-inflammatory treatments are being used for eczema. The type of emollient you need will differ according to things like your age and your skin type, and there are loads to choose between. It can be difficult if you have eczema and are spot prone, but don't worry; there are lots of different types, some lighter than others, and we can generally find something that suits.

Manage inflammation (for eczema-prone skin)

Eczema can flare-up with no clear triggers, even if you're using regular emollients and avoiding anything that irritates your skin. This is because your skin is prone to inflammation, and your skin cells can react to the environment, stress, or even nothing at all! **Inflamed skin therefore needs managing as soon as it appears, with the right anti-inflammatory treatments used daily.** The most commonly used are topical corticosteroids and a topical immunomodulator called tacrolimus.

Steroids

There is understandably some confusion when we talk about using 'steroids' to treat eczema. There are a wide variety of steroids, all with different properties; the sex hormones (Chapter 3) and stress hormones are both types of steroid, as are the anabolic steroids that bodybuilders often use. We also have a group of anti-inflammatory steroids called corticosteroids which are the ones we use

> **Box 4.2** Guide to corticosteroids
>
> Topical corticosteroids have been shown to be effective and safe when used correctly, with very low risk of side effects.
>
> People do sometimes worry about the risks of putting steroids on their skin, but as with any other treatment it is important to balance these risks with potential benefits. Steroids can occasionally cause problems, if the wrong strength is used on the wrong areas of the body, for the wrong amount of time. We have a lot of evidence to reassure us that correct use of topical steroids in eczema is effective, however, and longer-term studies in eczema show no significant problems for people as they get older. The national guidelines, having examined all the evidence, state clearly that steroids can be very effective for inflamed eczema, and therefore that their benefits outweigh the harms when used correctly (Box 4.3).
>
> Despite this strong evidence, **research confirms that people often don't use enough topical corticosteroids; either that, or they use one that is too weak to control the skin due to concerns about the side effects of steroids.** Health workers are part of the problem, because pharmacists, GPs, and dermatologists might all advise and prescribe different things. In the dermatology clinic we often see bad eczema that is just due to people not using enough corticosteroid, or being confused about how and when to use it.

to treat eczema—they aren't going to help much with your bodybuilding, as these are a totally different class of steroids from the ones you hear being used to build muscles in (cheating) athletes (Box 4.2).

Alternatives to steroid ointments

Calcineurin inhibitors (tacrolimus and pimecrolimus) can be alternative anti-inflammatory treatments (Chapter 11). They may not be as effective as topical steroids for areas on the body but are useful in delicate areas like eyelids or face where steroid ointments could possibly cause problems or may not be able to control eczema. Some people find they sting or burn when you first use them and this often settles down. Topical calcineurin inhibitors have been used for over 20 years to manage eczema. Studies over this time seems to show they are both effective and safe however there is ongoing monitoring to assess any potential long-term risks.

Get control and keep control

Evidence now shows that it is better to get control of the eczema with a stronger corticosteroid, rather than to keep trying with ineffective weaker ones. Enough needs to be applied to the skin to work, as this is a medicine; rubbing a tiny amount into lots of skin is the same as expecting a crumb of paracetamol to cure a bad headache. Applying on top of a thick layer of emollient is also not going to be effective. You need to put enough steroid on to leave your skin 'glistening'. After a few weeks of this the inflamed eczema should be controlled, and then it can be kept that way with regular 'proactive' or 'weekend' treatments. This involves putting the treatment on to flare-prone areas, such as the creases of your arms, or your face even when the eczema does not look or feel active. The skin may appear completely normal, but we know that the cells there are ready to flare-up with any, or even no, excuse. By targeting these areas with an anti-inflammatory cream (either a topical steroid or tacrolimus), you can manage this 'background' inflammation (Box 4.3). Studies have shown this is both a safe and effective way of preventing flares. Some people can use this technique for some months, and if the eczema stops flaring-up they may not need to continue. This may well control the condition for a while, but eczema likely will flare-up again. If this happens, don't panic. Just restart the treatments needed to control things.

Keep things simple. Find one emollient you like and use to wash and if skin feels dry. Get one active treatment for face and one for body and use daily when bad and at weekends to control if needed. Taking responsibility for your own treatment can help. Most young people do not want their parents putting creams and ointments on and this is great (although you may need some help for places you can't reach) (Fig. 4.3).

Box 4.3 'Steroid withdrawal syndrome'/SWS

Some people have suggested that eczema actually responds abnormally to steroid use, and can become inflamed if too much steroid is used or if steroids are stopped all of a sudden. This theoretical condition has been named 'steroid withdrawal syndrome'. The idea is that if this happens, steroids should be stopped entirely, and the skin should just be left to go through this process of inflammation until it finally settles. There are some advocates for this, including a few medical professionals, but currently there is not much good evidence and this likely covers several different issues. While research is ongoing we would simply advise using evidence-based approaches to managing your eczema, which will ensure you're using topical steroids appropriately.

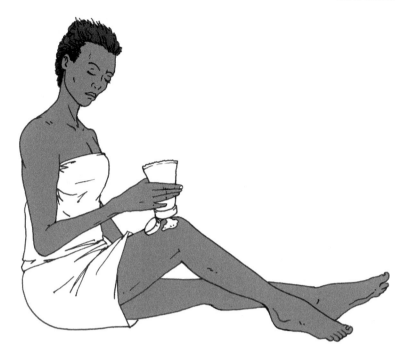

Figure 4.3 Steroid ointments are safe and effective when used to manage eczema.
© Reproduced courtesy of Damian Hale.

Itch in eczema

Inflammation makes eczema very itchy and this can have a massive effect on many aspects of life, especially sleep and concentration. Scratching is pretty unavoidable if skin is itchy but further damages the barrier of the skin, increases the inflammation, and can get into a bad cycle. Managing eczema well can reduce itch and help. Addressing a cycle of itch/scratch can be important especially if you find you are still scratching when eczema seems well controlled (Box 4.4).

Infections in eczema

All of us go through everyday life with a vast number of bugs—including bacteria, yeasts, and fungi—on our skin (Chapter 14). The majority of these are totally normal, but we do find that there are certain bugs more likely to survive on skin prone to eczema. Often this just reflects the fact that the eczema needs

Box 4.4 Itching and scratching

Most of your bodily organs can cause you to feel pain, but your skin is the only organ that can feel itchy. Itch is a really distracting and unpleasant sensation, which causes you to want to rub or scratch at your skin. Occasionally it's useful; if something bites you, for example, you'll realize it's itching and flick it off. More often however, it is a result of inflammatory processes in the skin, and in this case the itch will be far less helpful. Common conditions such as eczema, scabies, and fungal infection all lead to activation in complicated pathways involved in itch, often with irritating results.

Scratching might feel really good, at least for a short time. It turns the itch into a pain instead, which can seem much better at first. The problem is that once you scratch, you cause further inflammation that will in turn make the itch worse. This is called the 'itch-scratch cycle'. You may already have noticed that areas of the body you can't reach so well—like the middle of your back, for example—have fewer scratches on them, and therefore are less inflamed as a result.

It's impossible to ignore itch, so just being told not to scratch is usually pretty unhelpful. Thankfully, there are other things you can do that might be useful;

- Make sure your nails are short and blunt, so that even if you scratch—which you might do without realizing—you won't be able to damage your skin so much.

- Try to avoid skin getting dry and irritated; avoid soaps, and instead use moisturizers that make skin more 'slippy' and less easily broken. Sometimes cooling the moisturizer before use can help, or choosing a moisturizer that contains menthol in order to provide the same cooling effect.

- Try not to get too hot—especially at night—as this will make you even itchier.

- Treat the cause of your itch as effectively as possible. This is probably the most important part, and the chapters covering the treatment of eczema, infection, and urticaria should help!

Itching can become a habit, which can make it difficult to break the 'itch-scratch cycle'. You might just be rubbing your neck or fingers together when you're nervous, for example, and so habit reversal (Chapter 17) could be useful if you're itching a lot without realizing.

to be managed better, but sometimes these bugs can cause infections that make the skin even more inflamed.

One particular example is a bacterium called staphylococcal aureus (sometimes just referred to as staph), which has the potential to make both atopic and discoid eczema worse. Staph becomes less of a problem in eczema if we are able to reduce how inflamed the skin is however, so the **most important thing to do is manage the inflammation with anti-inflammatory treatments** (Box 4.2). Overuse of antibiotics in eczema is a big problem, and many people—including the World Health Organization (WHO)—feel they are often given inappropriately. We advise simply trying to reduce how inflamed the eczema is and using techniques to eliminate the effect of staph on the process. This could be achieved by using an emollient cream with antiseptic in it for example, or even by adding bleach to your bath every so often (half a cup once a week). The evidence isn't currently clear as to whether this really reduces bugs on the skin, or in fact just helps the skin's barrier function; either way it seems to work for some people. This might sound ridiculous but is really pretty similar to swimming pool water—which can also be a good antiseptic for your skin.

Yeasts can also cause similar problems in a specific type of eczema called seborrheic eczema. This condition affects the 'seborrheic' areas, which are the parts of the body that have more sebaceous glands. These produce an oily substance that coats your skin, and lots of them are found on the scalp—where they can cause dandruff—and around the eyebrows. Certain yeasts called *Malassezia* seem to thrive in these areas, and are likely to be part of the issue; treatment may therefore require both an anti-inflammatory and a medication to reduce the growth of yeast, which can often be given in the form of a shampoo.

There are other infections that are common in the general population, but may be worse in people with eczema including warts and molluscum (Chapter 14). Fungal infections like athlete's foot don't seem to be more common, but can look like eczema; we therefore need to be careful that the diagnosis is right, as the treatment is very different.

Eczema herpeticum

People with atopic eczema are more vulnerable to a serious infection caused by the same virus that gives people cold sores, known as herpes simplex virus (HSV). HSV infection can spread more widely in eczema, and it has the potential to make you feel unwell. This infection—which causes little blisters or sores on the skin—is seen more commonly in people with severe eczema, and needs medical assessment and urgent treatment.

If you feel unwell and your eczema skin seems crusty, oozy, and particularly if there are small blisters and sores then you do need to see a doctor. They may do swabs and consider treatments for secondary infection.

Why treat symptoms of eczema rather than trying to find the cause?

It may feel frustrating to just be controlling your symptoms, rather than getting to the cause of atopic eczema. Remember that the causes of eczema are complex; 'curing' people is not really possible, but eczema will still often seem to disappear with the 'get control, keep control' regime.

It is worth trying to get on top of eczema. Sometimes young people understandably have had enough and do not want to engage with any treatments and say they would rather just 'live with it' and just want everyone to stop bothering them.

Firstly, it doesn't have to be too much effort and secondly sometimes you don't realize how much your eczema was bothering you until it is improved.

Eczema can feel like an annoying, complicated condition to live with, but the management can be really quite simple.

Eczema shouldn't stop you living your life

Eczema should not stop you being who you want and doing what you want. Many patients carry on regardless even when their skin is bad but some do end up avoiding and missing things even when their skin is OK. Hopefully by understanding and managing your eczema better this will help. There will be some days when it is all too much your skin is sore, you feel rubbish, or you are just too busy to deal with your skin—that's OK too. If your eczema is getting you down, or life is getting you down, do talk or find someone to help you.

Other treatments for eczema

Sometimes eczema cannot be controlled easily with topical treatments and a few patients do need tablets or injections to control things long term. These are exciting times for eczema. There is still no 'cure' but there are recent advances in scientific understanding. These are leading to better use of treatments in more targeted ways and development of many novel treatments which are now available for severe eczema (Chapter 8). There is also better understanding of how eczema can affect all aspects of life in adolescence and hopefully better support available.

Resources

Ichthyosis (very dry, scaly skin)
Ichthyosis support group. Excellent resource for patients of all ages with ichthyosis:
> http://www.ichthyosis.org.uk

Eczema
Young people's experiences of eczema:
> http://healthtalk.org/young-peoples-experiences/eczema/topics

Website for National Eczema Society (NES) Information booklet 'Teenagers with Eczema—live your life' available on website:
> http://eczema.org/

Eczema Outreach Support (EOS)—A national organisation providing support for families, children and young people living with eczema:
> https://ww.eos.org.uk

Nottingham centre for evidence-based dermatology have lots of excellent patient resources:
> http://www.nottinghameczema.org.uk/information/index.aspx

Information for teenagers with eczema:
> http://www.nottinghameczema.org.uk/documents/teenage-eczema.pdf

Get Control and Keep Control: Oxford University Hospitals information:
> https://www.ouh.nhs.uk/patient-guide/leaflets/files/5608Pcontrol.pdf

Graphic image on topical Get Control and Keep Control:
> http://www.nottinghameczema.org.uk/documents/eczemaposter2020.pdf
> https://www.skinhealthinfo.org.uk/national-eczema-society-and-british-association-of-dermatologists-joint-position-statement-on-topical-steroid-withdrawal/

5

Hives/Urticaria

 Key points

- Hives—also known as urticaria—are itchy bumps that sometimes appear on the skin for a short time.

- There are many causes of urticaria, other than just allergy—having hives does not necessarily mean that you're allergic to something.

- The most common form of urticaria is spontaneous urticaria, where a trigger is never found. If this continues for a long time, however, the cause may be autoimmune.

- Antihistamines are generally an effective treatment to control urticaria; the long-acting, non-sedating versions are usually best.

What is urticaria?

Urticaria is the medical name for hives, which are also known as either wheals or 'nettle rash'. These are itchy marks that appear suddenly on the skin, with a well-defined red edge and pale, swollen area at the centre. Typically, an individual hive will clear within 24 hours, although the overall rash may well last longer; occasionally they cause bruising—especially if scratched—but the majority should just leave normal skin behind. If they last longer than 24–48 hours then they might not actually be hives, and alternative causes such as acute eczema should be considered.

Angioedema is a form of urticaria in which there is deeper swelling in the skin. This may be around the eyes, lips, or genitals, or sometimes elsewhere on the body. The swelling is less itchy, but can be more painful, and it may take longer than 24 hours to settle.

The main symptom of urticaria is itch, which can potentially be really distressing. Feeling itchy, often at unpredictable times, can have a big impact

Skin Conditions in Young People. Tess McPherson, Oxford University Press. © Oxford University Press 2021.
DOI: 10.1093/oso/9780192895424.003.0005

on your sleep; combined with the effect of urticaria on your skin's appearance, it can cause significant changes to your overall quality of life too. Angioedema tends not to be as itchy, but that doesn't mean people find it any less unpleasant, however. Rarely, the swelling caused by angioedema may affect the tongue or throat, leading to difficulty breathing or swallowing; this can be alarming for patients, although thankfully it is rarely life-threatening.

Urticaria and angioedema appear when cells in the skin—known as mast cells—suddenly release a load of chemicals, including one called histamine. If someone is allergic to something, these mast cells might be triggered by the thing they are allergic too; a food, for example, or maybe drugs, dusts, pollens, and wasp or bee stings. By far the most common form is 'spontaneous urticaria' however, for which there is no clear trigger. In spontaneous urticaria, the release of histamine is not due to allergy, but instead due to factors that make the mast cells more reactive. Acute spontaneous urticaria lasts less than 6 weeks, and is often due to a minor infection, whereas chronic urticaria lasts longer than this.

Allergy and urticaria

Urticaria and angioedema usually develop very quickly if the cause is allergic. The rash and swelling happen very quickly in response to allergens, usually within minutes, and this can be very scary and needs urgent treatment. An allergy specialist can help to identify the cause, and if it sounds like you do have an allergy to something, there will be carefully selected allergy tests that can be arranged. The allergy—particularly if it is a food allergy—tends to appear at an early age. As discussed in the section on eczema, these types of immediate reactions to food are much less likely to develop newly in adolescence. Medicines can also cause acute urticaria, and almost any drug can be responsible. Painkillers like aspirin and ibuprofen, as well as antibiotics—particularly those containing penicillins—are the common culprits. As long as you know what causes the allergy however, avoiding it will prevent the reactions from happening.

If you already know you have a food allergy, adolescence can be a tricky time. You are eating away from home more, and it can be less easy to avoid hidden foods like nuts, egg, cow's milk, and sesame. Labelling is getting better, but make sure you check ingredients of any food carefully each time. You don't always have to avoid foods labelled as 'may contain' or 'traces of' unless you have been advised to by your healthcare specialist, but you can always ask them if you're not sure. Also remember that kissing someone who has just eaten a food you are allergic to—for example nuts—can occasionally be risky, and they won't necessarily come with a label!

Make sure that you carry your adrenaline autoinjector—brand names include EpiPen, Jext, or Emerade—at all times, as these can be life-saving if you do develop a reaction.

Most hives are not caused by allergy

As mentioned previously, the most common cause of urticaria is spontaneous urticaria. In this condition the hives can come and go at any point in the day or night, and are not related to any clear trigger. Some activities may make flares worse: exercise, heat, alcohol, painkillers such as ibuprofen, emotion, and even your periods can exacerbate things. Whatever the cause, the episodes can be very annoying. Fortunately, urticaria tends to resolve, although it can take a few months; rarely, chronic urticaria can last up to 10 to 20 years!

Physical triggers can also cause urticaria, and these forms of urticaria have specific names:

- Dermographism—caused by scratching the skin
- Delayed pressure urticaria—caused by pressure on the skin
- Solar urticaria—triggered by sunlight
- Aquagenic urticaria—caused by water
- Cold urticaria
- Cholinergic urticaria

These are all types of chronic inducible urticaria (CIndU). **Cholinergic urticaria** is pretty common in young people and can be triggered by sweat, heat, hot showers, emotional stress, and spicy food. It causes very small hives to appear within minutes, usually on the upper part of the body, although they can be widespread. The rash generally lasts for less than 1 hour, but—especially if it seems to be triggered by emotional situations—can feel embarrassing. As it isn't triggered by an allergen, no allergy tests are needed for this type of urticaria. Fortunately, cholinergic urticaria normally responds well to antihistamine treatments (see next), especially before a known triggering event such as exercise.

Why me?

Urticaria very common, and at least 1 in 5 people will experience an episode of spontaneous urticaria at some point in their lives. The clue is in the name; this often happens spontaneously, with no clear trigger or reason behind it. It seems likely that there are things that can make mast cells more reactive; infections such as a cold, sore throat, or the flu may act as a trigger, for instance. Some people also have an inherited tendency to autoimmune conditions, for example, and this may also make urticaria more likely.

When do I need tests?

If the urticaria happens immediately—within less than an hour of a possible trigger—then an allergy is more likely. You will probably be referred to the allergy clinic, for skin and blood tests to look for the cause. It's worth knowing that most people do not need any tests, however, as they will not be able to identify an allergic cause or change the suggested treatment.

An urticarial rash may rarely be associated with a fever, joint pains, or stiffness, bruising, or feeling unwell; this can be a sign of underlying health conditions, and so you should speak to a doctor about this.

Management of urticaria

The first—and most obvious—thing to do is to try to avoid anything that worsens your urticaria, such as heat, tight clothes, medications, and alcohol. Avoidance of specific foods, colouring agents, and preservatives is only helpful in the rare instances where these have proven to be a problem.

Treatments for urticaria

Antihistamines block the effect of histamine, the chemical released by mast cells. This can therefore reduce itching and the rash in most people, but may not relieve urticaria completely. If urticaria occurs frequently, it is best to take antihistamines regularly each day. There are many different types of non-sedating and sedating antihistamines, which are both available as either short-acting or long-acting versions. In general, the once-a-day, long-acting, non-sedating antihistamines are the best; examples include cetirizine, loratadine, and fexofenadine. The first two can be bought over the counter, whereas fexofenadine has to be prescribed by a doctor. Your doctor may need to try different ones, and can increase the doses as necessary to find a regime that suits you best; doses can be increased above that recommended on the packet if needs be, but you should discuss this with a doctor beforehand. The antihistamine tablets can be taken for as long as the urticaria persists, and you can always restart them if you need to.

If your urticaria is not controlled by antihistamines, an antiasthma tablet is sometimes also used. Tablets called cimetidine and ranitidine, which are usually used to treat stomach ulcers, can also be added to the standard antihistamines if urticaria persists or is resistant to treatment. Oral steroids might occasionally be given briefly for a few days in severe flares of acute and chronic urticaria, but generally are not necessary.

Most people can control their symptoms by taking these treatments regularly. For the most severely affected people—who don't respond to these—there are other treatments available that act by suppressing the immune system. These include ciclosporin (Chapter 8) and a drug called omalizumab; omalizumab is given every month via injection, and works very well in most people.

Very rarely, injections of adrenaline may be required to reverse breathing problems, which can occur with angioedema. If you are having problems with breathing or swallowing you need to get urgent medical advice, as rapid treatment may be necessary.

The treatments discussed in this chapter will suppress your condition rather than cure it, but over time it should disappear. Urticaria gradually resolves in most people over 1–2 years, and you can adjust the treatments according to how much you need them over this time. It is a bit unpredictable, and can last considerably longer in some people, but there are a variety of treatments on offer to help control the symptoms.

Resources

British Association of Dermatologists patient information:

> https://www.bad.org.uk/for-the-public/patient-information-leaflets/urticaria-and-angioedema

6

Psoriasis

 Key points

- Psoriasis affects 1–2% of the population.

- It can develop at any age, but quite often comes on in people's teens or twenties.

- Psoriasis might not involve just the skin, as it can affect other body parts as well.

- There are plenty of treatments to help manage and control psoriasis, and so having psoriasis shouldn't stop you from doing whatever you want to.

What is psoriasis?

Psoriasis is due to inflammation in the skin (like eczema but slightly different bunch of inflammatory cells) (Box 2.1). Psoriasis is not contagious and cannot be 'caught'. It is pretty common and affects around 1–2% of the population. It can develop at any age—from infancy through to adulthood—but the most common time for it to come on is in the teens and twenties.

There are several different types of psoriasis, but two are more common in younger people:

Chronic plaque psoriasis: This is the most common type. Chronic means the symptoms can come and go at any time throughout life. Areas of the body most often affected are the scalp—in particular behind ears—the elbows and knees, the navel area (around the belly button), and the genital area. Psoriasis varies from person to person, both in severity and how it responds to treatment. There is unfortunately no cure for psoriasis, but there are many treatment options available to help; the specific type used will depend both on how bad the psoriasis is, and where it's located on the body.

Skin Conditions in Young People. Tess McPherson, Oxford University Press. © Oxford University Press 2021.
DOI: 10.1093/oso/9780192895424.003.0006

Guttate psoriasis: Small areas of psoriasis mostly on trunk which typically appear just after a throat infection. This may happen as a one-off episode, but can occur repeatedly in some people. It might also make it more likely that you will develop chronic plaque psoriasis.

Why me?

We don't know exactly what causes psoriasis, but both inherited and environmental factors play a role in its development. The reason we think the genes we inherit are involved is that it tends to run in families; if one parent has the condition then there is a 25% chance that their child will also have it, and the odds go up to 40% if both parents have psoriasis.

That said it's a complicated process, and it seems there are things in the environments we live in that can trigger the development of psoriasis too. Injury to the skin, common colds, and throat infections, certain medications; these all tend to cause psoriasis to flare up in younger people, especially those who were already predisposed to the condition.

We think the reason that injuries and infections trigger 'flare-ups' of psoriasis is that they activate the immune system, the defence your body normally uses to fix these kinds of problems. In patients with psoriasis, the immune system is inappropriately activated, however, which results in faster turnover of skin cells. Usually, the skin is constantly renewing and healing itself, shedding the outer layer of skin cells while new ones are made underneath. Each skin cell generally lasts about 3–4 weeks before it falls off, but in psoriasis they can take just 3–4 days to go through this cycle. They therefore pile up instead of falling off, forming thickened, scaly patches (Fig. 6.1).

What does psoriasis look like?

Psoriasis can be widespread or localized to elbows, knees, scalp and in between buttocks (Fig. 6.2). Why psoriasis likes these areas is not well understood, but given that scratches can cause psoriasis, it could partly be down to the fact that we get more friction in those places. Patches of psoriasis are demarcated, which means it's easy to see the boundary between the patch of psoriasis and the skin around it and have thick almost 'silvery' scale.

Chronic plaque psoriasis is also more likely to cause changes in fingernails and toenails. They can grow thicker, or sometimes develop little dimples known as 'pits'. Your joints may be affected too, becoming painful, swollen, and making them difficult to move. Psoriasis is thought to be associated with a few other

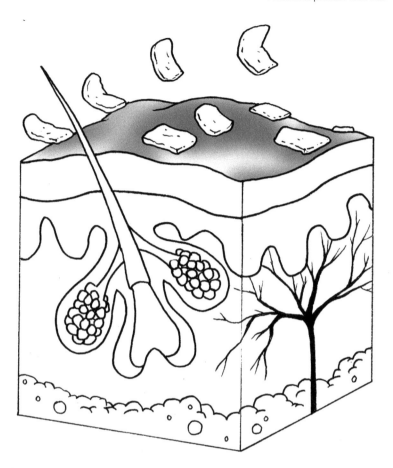

Figure 6.1 Psoriasis skin cells are active, causing inflammation and scale.
© Reproduced courtesy of Damian Hale.

health conditions as well as these, which often appear later in life; we'll talk a bit more about this later.

All the changes psoriasis causes will understandably affect how you feel about yourself. The flaky skin can feel embarrassing. Some people describe themselves as 'ashamed' or 'dirty', which then makes them scared to expose their skin. This might lead to them avoiding certain activities, becoming increasingly anxious or low in mood. Mental health can therefore take a big hit in psoriasis

49

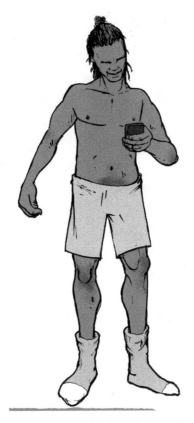

Figure 6.2 Chronic plaque psoriasis usually affects elbows and knees, belly button, and groin area.
© Reproduced courtesy of Damian Hale.

too, and so there are two important things to remember; the first is that it's not your fault, and the second is that there are lots of treatments that can help.

Treatments for psoriasis

Unfortunately, there is no cure for chronic plaque psoriasis. The word chronic doesn't necessarily mean that it's serious, just that it lasts a long time. It can obviously be depressing to hear that your psoriasis is most likely going to be a life-long thing, but this doesn't mean that it can't be controlled or has to be a problem. There are plenty of effective treatments that can help reduce symptoms and make it less problematic, so having psoriasis should not stop you living your life to the full.

Treatments will either be 'topical' options that are applied to the skin, or 'systemic' treatments that aim to treat the whole body at once; tablets, injections, and light therapy are all examples of these.

Topical treatments

The first and easiest step is to start using an emollient. This is essentially a fancy name for a moisturizer, and will help if your skin feels dry or flaky. You can use any moisturizer that you find suits you, as people with psoriasis generally don't need to be as careful with fragranced products as those with sensitive skin or eczema do.

Active treatments can then be added on top of this, in an attempt to reduce scaling and inflammation of the skin. Many of these are not specifically licensed for use in people under the age of 18, but are still safe, well-tested, and routinely prescribed. They include **corticosteroids**, **vitamin D analogues**, **dithranol**, and **tacrolimus**, all of which come in various forms; you will be able to find them as either ointments, gels, or foams, and they can be used alone or in combination. Different treatments work better on different areas of the skin, so your doctor should tell you what to use where. They are applied as needed to the affected areas and, other than a few exceptions, aren't normally required if things are under control.

Topical treatments can manage psoriasis very well for a lot of people, although it is still likely that areas will flare up occasionally. It might also seem as if your psoriasis has stopped responding to treatments that have previously worked, at which point it's worth discussing what else is available. There are always plenty more options to choose from, and you could consider revisiting things that have helped in the past.

Treating specific areas

The scalp

The scalp is often affected in psoriasis, and your hair can therefore make treating this area slightly tricky. In this case, we find it helpful to consider treating scale and treating inflammation separately. This can usually be achieved by applying something to the scalp overnight that will reduce the scale, before using a comb the next morning to lift it off. A separate treatment—either a shampoo or a scalp lotion—can then be applied to help with the redness and itch caused by inflammation.

This can feel like a bit of a project, but it's worth giving things a good go. Choosing a time when you have a few days that you can devote to it can work well. It should then be easier to keep your psoriasis under control after this, just using treatments every so often from then on.

Genital psoriasis

Psoriasis can quite commonly affect the area of skin around the genitals, particularly the bit in between the buttocks. People often don't feel comfortable telling their doctors about this, and some health professionals may not think to ask; it's important to address though, because it might mean you are more likely to have the type of psoriasis that can cause joint problems too. Even if you don't, the skin can still become a big issue, so make sure to discuss the treatments available.

Systemic treatments

If your psoriasis is particularly bad, spread out, or difficult to control with creams and gels, then other treatments may be considered.

Light treatment

If quite a lot of skin is affected by psoriasis, then something called ultraviolet (UV) phototherapy can be used. This involves shining UV light onto the skin in an attempt to reduce the inflammation. You may have noticed that natural sunlight can improve your skin, although sadly people with psoriasis don't tend to expose their skin as much; it helps because sunlight contains many different types of UV light, and it's the same idea behind this treatment.

Too much sunlight can result in sunburn, however, increasing the risk of wrinkling, skin cancer, and even new psoriasis. UV therapy therefore only uses a specific type of UV light, called narrow band UVB. This seems to be the best at reducing inflammation in the skin, while it also has the lowest risk of early skin ageing and skin cancer.

The light treatments are normally given in the hospital, and happen three times a week for about 4–5 months. This means it might not be ideal if you live far away from the hospital, or have school, college, or a job that is difficult to work around. Sunbeds or home treatments are not so safe, as it's not as easy to keep track of how much light you've had in total. They also sometimes use other types of UV light—such as UVA—that come with a higher risk of skin damage. It's important to monitor these things, because there is a certain amount of light treatment that is agreed to be safe in a lifetime. It's therefore not suitable as a continuous treatment, and if you have very fair skin or a family history of skin cancer then it might not be suitable at all.

Light treatment can be brilliant for some people. How long the effects last is really variable; guttate psoriasis can be totally cured by a single course of UVB, and chronic plaque psoriasis may stay clear for years following light treatment. Frustratingly, other people's psoriasis can come back almost as soon as they have finished the course, in which case other treatments should be considered.

Tablets and injections

We mentioned previously that psoriasis might be caused by an overactive immune system, and so a lot of the systemic treatments—both tablets and injections—target the way your immune system works. They therefore need regular blood tests and reviews, in order to watch out for side effects.

Methotrexate is the most commonly used systemic medication for psoriasis, and there is a lot of evidence that it can be safe and effective for a long time in some people. Other options include *acitretin* and *ciclosporin*, which can both be equally as useful.

If these treatments don't work, or cause too many side effects, there are now newer medications given by injection called biologics available. These can be very effective for severe psoriasis, but will also need to be regularly monitored. With any of these options, you always have to consider the benefits and possible risks—you can read more about this in Chapter 8 on systemic treatments.

Psoriasis and other health problems

There is increasing evidence that in some cases, particularly if psoriasis is severe, it's not just the skin that will be affected. This kind of thing is seen in a lot of conditions that involve inflammation—including eczema, for example—but psoriasis has some of the strongest links to inflammation in other parts of the body. The joints, the liver, and the heart may all be affected, and there's also a potential link with obesity. Why this happens is not completely clear though. We're trying to work out how inflammation in the skin affects other body parts, and whether the treatments we currently prescribe for psoriasis will help these other body parts too.

Although psoriasis is not caused by being unhealthy, keeping active and staying at a healthy weight are really important. Exercise has been shown to reduce how severe psoriasis can be, and may even lessen the chances of getting psoriasis in the first place. It's therefore a massive help, both right now and in the future; given that we think people with psoriasis might be at greater risk of conditions like heart disease and obesity, it will hopefully reduce the odds of developing these too. We see lots of patients who don't want to expose their skin, which means they tend to shy away from swimming or other sports. It's hard, but try to find any way you can to keep active; it will likely make you feel better at the same time.

We know that having a skin condition like psoriasis when you are young can have a big say in how you feel about yourself. Make sure you get psychological support if you need it, to help work out how you can keep psoriasis from having a negative impact on your life both now and in the future.

It's OK to have a bit of psoriasis on your skin. It might be tempting to think that the only way you could enjoy your life is if it went away, but getting on with it and not being so hard on yourself might actually be the best way to go.

Resources

Young people's experiences of Psoriasis:

> http://healthtalk.org/young-peoples-experiences/psoriasis/topics

Specific UK website targeting teenagers and young people with psoriasis:

> https://www.psoteen.org.uk

American website for psoriasis and psoriatic arthritis:

> https://www.psoriasis.org/for-teens/

British Association of Dermatology patient information:

> https://www.skinhealthinfo.org.uk/condition/psoriasis-in-children-and-young-people/
> https://www.skinhealthinfo.org.uk/condition/psoriasis/
> https://www.skinhealthinfo.org.uk/condition/topical-treatments-for-psoriasis/
> https://www.skinhealthinfo.org.uk/condition/phototherapy-nb-uvb/

7

Hidradenitis suppurativa

What is hidradenitis suppurativa?

Hidradenitis suppurativa—sometimes just abbreviated to HS—involves inflammation of glands in the skin. These glands are called apocrine glands, and most of them are found in the armpits, groin, and breasts. For reasons we don't fully understand, in HS these glands behave abnormally; they are more prone to becoming blocked and inflamed, which can cause skin problems similar to those seen in acne. HS actually used to be called acne inversa for this reason, as it leads to comedones and pus-filled abscesses (more commonly called blackheads and boils). HS is a common condition that affects between 0.4 and 4% of the population in UK, and is most likely to develop in young adults. The numbers might even be higher than that, as we know that many people are not correctly diagnosed or do not seek appropriate help. It is a chronic condition, by which we mean it is a long-term thing that gets better and worse over time.

Why me?

HS is a complex condition, and the causes are not completely understood. As with other inflammatory skin conditions, however (Box 2.1), both your genes and the environment that you live in play a role. If someone in your family has

HS, for example, then you are probably more prone to it too; about a third of people with the condition will have a relative that has HS as well. Certain things are clearly shown to increase the risk of developing HS—such as being overweight and smoking—but it can certainly be seen in underweight people, and even those who have never smoked a cigarette in their life.

HS is not contagious, and is not related to poor hygiene. Deodorant will therefore neither cause nor prevent it. Although patients can often develop different skin infections if they have HS, it is not because they are any dirtier than anybody else.

What are glands?

When people refer to their 'glands being up' they are generally talking about something called their lymph nodes, which are centres of immune response. These nodes are in groups, around your neck, for example, and get big and sore when the immune system is dealing with, for instance, an infection. The medical definition of glands is slightly different: collections of cells that produce various substances, which they are then able to release. There are a few types of glands in the skin, which secrete various substances; the sebaceous glands produce oil for example, and are involved in acne, whereas eccrine glands are responsible for sweating. Apocrine glands (Fig. 7.1) are the ones that cause the problem in HS, and their role is a bit more complicated.

Apocrine glands

As babies we have apocrine glands all over the skin, before they settle in certain areas after we've grown. The armpits, breast, groin, ears, and eyelids are where most are eventually found. They don't do much before puberty, but at this point hormonal changes make them larger and busier. This is probably why some female patients find that HS flares up when they're on their period, as these hormones are playing their role.

Your apocrine glands secrete smelly substances, sometimes called pheromones, which are supposed to attract other humans. They can be activated by plenty of different hormones, including adrenaline, for example. This is released when we're in pain, stressed, frightened, or even having sex, and might therefore cause your apocrine glands to be working at those times too. They won't just give out pheromones however, because they've got a few other uses—apocrine glands secrete a thick clear fluid in the ears that can help you make earwax, and in breasts they secrete milk.

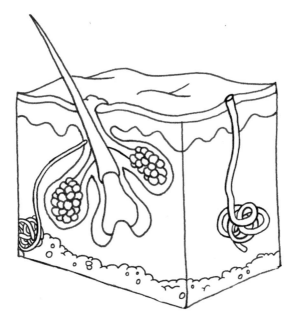

Figure 7.1 Apocrine glands in skin opens into hair follicle. In HS these become inflamed.
© Reproduced courtesy of Damian Hale.

Apocrine glands in hidradenitis suppurativa

The problems in HS seem to begin with the blockage of apocrine glands. This allows things to build up, causing inflammation that eventually leads to painful spots in the skin (Fig. 7.2). These might then discharge pus, or even become infected if bacteria get trapped there too.

The spots usually appear in areas of the skin that aren't often exposed, and so HS can be a hidden disease. Research shows people might just try to cope, not wanting to see their doctor about it, and that even if they do seek medical attention it can take years for a correct diagnosis to be made. Although it often gets confused with acne, it is a separate condition. The process by which spots appear is admittedly quite similar, and people with bad acne can be prone to HS, but it is still a different diagnosis that shouldn't be missed.

There are several other conditions that seem to be related to HS, including one called pilonidal sinus that also causes abscesses to form. Other examples, such as a bowel condition known as Crohn's disease, or the skin condition psoriasis,

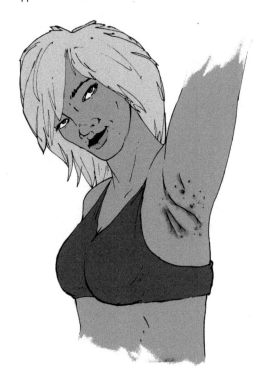

Figure 7.2 Hidradenitis in armpit.
© Reproduced courtesy of Damian Hale.

should also make doctors think about whether HS might be an issue for these patients too.

What happens in hidradenitis suppurativa?

If you have HS then you know that flares ups can be very painful, and the skin lesions are usually sore to the touch. They might just start as blackheads and small boils, but often become quite large. Discharge of pus can be a problem, and so they may require daily dressings, plus the areas of broken skin can get further infections if bacteria can then enter through them.

In the later stages, tunnels under the skin sometimes form, connecting boils or sores and therefore making it difficult for them to heal. The process may even cause scarring, which can become more extensive over time if flare-ups keep happening. It might settle down, but permanent scars are a possibility.

Patients with HS are therefore incredibly brave, and often tolerate an amazing amount of pain and discomfort. It can have a massive impact on so many things—the way you feel about your body in particular—and might then affect the intimate relationships you have with other people as a result.

Smoking in hidradenitis suppurativa

Why smoking triggers HS in certain people is a bit of a mystery. It seems that something in cigarettes affects certain cells in the skin, particularly the immune cells known as neutrophils that form pus. It's possible that the actual nicotine in cigarettes is to blame, as vaping appears to be associated with HS too. Either way it's an important trigger in the initiation of HS, so not starting to smoke is the best thing to do. Giving up smoking if you've already got HS might help, and it will be good for your heart and your lungs too, but remember it's much easier to never start in the first place.

Weight in hidradenitis suppurativa

Although being overweight is not the one thing that causes HS, there is no doubt that being or becoming overweight has a role in triggering and making HS worse. This might partly be due to increased friction in areas like the armpits and groin, which could then contribute to blocking skin pores and increasing inflammation.

We all know that losing weight is easier said than done. Exercise can feel impossible when you have painful, active flare-ups, or oozing areas of skin. Despite this, it is really worth trying to address; you can take control in deciding what you eat, and trying to keep as active as possible. Walking is good if anything more strenuous feels difficult. Keeping a healthy weight is really important, not just because it will help HS, but in keeping you healthy too.

What can I do?

Management of hidradenitis suppurativa

If you do have HS, trying to keep a healthy weight and steering clear of cigarettes are important, positive things that you can do. Avoiding tight clothes, which may increase friction to the skin, can be helpful too. There is also some evidence that laser pubic hair removal might be better than shaving or waxing the pubic area, but this is unfortunately not something everyone can afford.

Although there is no cure for HS, there are plenty of treatments that can be offered on top of the aforementioned suggestions. In the earlier stages of HS these will usually be options such as gels and tablets, whereas more longstanding and severe HS could benefit from operations. There is no cure for HS, but treatments such as these can be very effective in both preventing and treating flare-ups. They can't switch off HS once and for all, but it may become inactive eventually.

Basic steps

Lots of patients have their own way of dealing with things when they experience an acute flare. Warm baths and clean flannels can be helpful in getting pus out of the skin, and washing with antiseptics may be useful in preventing bacterial infections from causing more problems. Smaller spots might benefit from treatment with an antibiotic gel called **clindamycin**, and tablet antibiotics may also be needed if you have an infection associated with a flare. The reason these are recommended is not because you are dirty, but simply due to certain bacteria being more commonly found on the skin once you develop HS.

Painkillers are also essential. You can buy basic options—like paracetamol and ibuprofen—over the counter, and these should help. People often put up with more pain than they should do though, so ask your doctor for an appropriate level of painkiller if you need to. They may not think to offer it otherwise.

Medical treatment to try to prevent flares

There are several tablet medications that have some evidence for use in HS. They may need to be used for long periods in order to prevent acute flares, or taken on-and-off for a few months at a time.

Antibiotic tablets can be used to suppress the inflammation involved in HS, rather than just to kill bacteria, in the same way they can be used for acne. A type of antibiotic called a tetracycline—such as lymecycline or doxycycline—is often tried initially, or alternatively a combination of two antibiotics, called clindamycin and rifampicin, might be used. These are strong antibiotics, and so they do have potential side effects; you might get an upset stomach, for example, or they could interact with your oral contraceptive pill to make it less effective. They are used at lower doses than we would prescribe for traditional 'infections', but they do still sometimes require regular blood tests to monitor things.

Retinoids—tablets related to vitamin A—can help in some patients. Isotretinoin is an example you might have heard mentioned before, as it is sometimes used to treat severe acne. It's sadly not as effective in HS. A different retinoid called acitretin seems to be better at stopping the blockages that occur in HS than other retinoids. Like isotretinoin, this can only be given by specialists in dermatology clinics, and similarly it's not really an option for younger woman who may want to have children in the next few years due to the harm it can do to unborn babies.

Hormone tablets known as antiandrogens may sometimes be useful for patients who experience flares of HS just before their periods, and can be given as part of a contraceptive pill.

Tablets to alter the immune system could also be considered, to try and improve HS by dampening down the inflammation. These include medicines such as dapsone and ciclosporin, and newer types—known as anti-TNFs—that are given as injections. Any medication that affects how your immune system works has potential risks however (see Chapter 8 on systemic treatments). This means regular blood tests are likely to be needed, and the benefits should be balanced against the potential side effects.

Surgical treatment

Acute, infected flares can sometimes require a visit to A + E, in order for spots or boils to be drained by a surgeon. Persistent discharge or inflammation in the same site might also benefit from surgery, especially if it isn't going away despite medical treatment. This may involve removing small areas of repeated inflammation, or a wider procedure to take away all the affected tissue. The bigger operations probably reduce the chance of HS coming back in the treated area when compared to smaller procedures, but healing times are generally longer. It's also worth noting that many surgeons will not agree to perform any operation if you are smoking.

More and more people who work in medicine are learning about HS, and luckily there is an increasing amount of research focusing on it currently. This is already leading to better understanding and treatment of the condition, but we still know getting the right support can be difficult. Patients may often know more than some health workers, and patient support groups can therefore be useful; there are good resources they can give you, so just make sure you ask for help if you need to.

Resources

British association of dermatology information:
> https://www.britishskinfoundation.org.uk/hidradenitis-suppurativa

Hidradenitis suparativa patient support:
> https://www.hstrust.org/

8

Oral and injection (systemic) treatments for inflammatory skin conditions

 Key points

- There are lots of treatments for chronic skin conditions that have good evidence to show they are effective.

- Many of these have potential side effects, and therefore require monitoring.

- The risks and benefits of medication will always be discussed with you.

- There are strict rules about how and when medicines can be prescribed, based on their effects, costs, and safety.

Systemic treatments

If inflammatory skin conditions such as eczema, psoriasis or hidradenitis suppurativa cannot be controlled with appropriate creams or ointments, there is occasionally a need for other medicines. Generally, these are either oral tablets, liquids, or sometimes injections. We call them systemic treatments because they can affect your entire body (to a certain degree), rather than just your skin. It's for this reason that light treatment is also put in the 'systemic' category; it treats all of your skin at once, which can be particularly useful in widespread psoriasis, for example.

Many of the medications in this chapter work to reduce unwanted inflammation in your skin, by targeting your immune system in order to reduce the

Skin Conditions in Young People. Tess McPherson, Oxford University Press. © Oxford University Press 2021.
DOI: 10.1093/oso/9780192895424.003.0008

amount of inflammation it causes. Retinoids are the one big exception to this rule, as they instead work by directly affecting how the skin functions.

For any systemic medication, potential benefits will have to be carefully considered against known or possible risks. When these medicines are new, there will have only been a short time to collect information about them before they start being used; for this reason, there exist national data collection systems that carefully monitor people taking systemic treatments. They continuously assess how well they work over time, and keep an eye out for any short- or long-term problems.

Oral steroids/prednisolone

We have talked about topical corticosteroids up to this point, and stressed that the benefits outweigh the risks when used to treat skin conditions correctly. Oral steroids such as prednisolone will also work for skin conditions, but because they're given as a tablet they will affect the entire body. This may help the skin, but used for longer periods can also lead to thinning of your bones, weight gain, and diabetes. They should therefore just be used for short courses, and only in specific circumstances when they are seriously needed.

Luckily there are lots of other systemic treatments mentioned next, which are safer and more effective in treating severe skin conditions over long periods.

Methotrexate

Methotrexate is a medication that targets many aspects of the immune system. It was originally used to treat cancer in the 1940s—and remains an important anticancer medicine—but it has also been used for a long time to treat inflammatory conditions. When given at much lower doses than used for cancer, it has been successful in treating rheumatoid arthritis, psoriatic arthritis, and many more besides. Dermatologists have used it to manage psoriasis for decades, and more recently it has been found to be helpful in severe eczema too.

Methotrexate does not have a licence for use in patients under the age of 18. This is unlikely to change sadly, as it would need a particular drug company to apply for one. It has been around for so long, and is made by so many different manufacturers, that nobody is interested in getting a licence at this stage. It can be prescribed 'off-licence', however, if a doctor believes that this would still be the best treatment for their patient. Methotrexate has been used for decades by many, many young people, has been shown to be safe, works well, and dermatologists are therefore experienced in using it to treat people under 18. For this reason, it is part of many national guidelines, and is often given to younger patients with skin conditions.

Methotrexate is given once a week, either as a tablet or an injection under the skin. It needs a bit of time to start working, and generally you won't see the impact until you've been taking it for a few months. You also have to take a vitamin called folic acid while on methotrexate, either once a week—on a different day to the one you take methotrexate—or on all the days you don't take methotrexate.

It works by affecting neutrophils—cells that form part of the immune system we need to fight infections—but this effect is not very specific. Most of the cells in your body are vulnerable to methotrexate, and so it does need to be monitored. You will have some 'baseline' blood tests before starting treatment, to check that your liver, your kidneys, and the cells in your blood are all OK, and you will need regular blood tests for the first few months too. Most serious problems occur early in treatment, so these are vital to keep you safe.

A common problem that young people report is nausea on the day they take their methotrexate, as well as feeling tired. Taking the methotrexate at weekends can help, and recent evidence shows that the nausea can be reduced by caffeine. If you like black coffee then just have one about an hour before taking the medicine, or dark chocolate will work just as well if you'd prefer that instead.

Alcohol should be avoided (or at least drunk as little as possible) while on methotrexate, as your liver is needed to process both of these substances and will struggle to deal with the two at once. You cannot have live vaccines—yellow fever, for example—while on treatment, so these should ideally be up to date before you start. Due to effects on growing cells it is also dangerous in pregnancy, and you should therefore be on reliable contraception when taking methotrexate.

Despite these cautions, many young people report little-to-no problems on methotrexate. It's an amazing drug, and is on the World Health Organization (WHO) list as one of the safest and most effective medicines needed in any health system. It is generally well tolerated, and can be used safely for many years as long as the correct blood tests are continued.

Ciclosporin

This medicine used to be used a lot for eczema; it does work quite quickly, for both eczema and psoriasis, and is safe in pregnancy so can be a good option for a short time. It's not a good drug to be on for a long time though, as it causes problems for your kidneys, plus it can increase the risk of cancer. Some patients have to be on a drug like ciclosporin—for instance, if they have had an organ transplant—and in this case the need outweighs the risk. Evidence shows that methotrexate is equally effective as ciclosporin for psoriasis or eczema, so if you are able to take either, then methotrexate is the safer option long term.

Azathioprine

This medication is another that used to be prescribed quite often, and can sometimes still be considered instead of methotrexate. There is data that suggests it might be associated with certain cancers—particularly skin cancers—if used for a long time however, so the risks and benefits will need to be carefully considered.

Retinoids: isotretinoin, acitretin, and alitretinoin

Retinoids are a class of drug related to vitamin A, and come in a few different forms: isotretinoin, acitretin, and alitretinoin are all types used to treat skin conditions.

Isotretinoin is a retinoid that affects the hair follicles, and also reduces the amount of grease produced by skin. It is therefore used to treat spots and acne (Chapter 3).

Acitretin and alitretinoin instead make the skin less scaly, by targeting a process called keratinization. Acitretin appears to work in a few different skin conditions; it is used for psoriasis, dermatitis (eczema) in the hands and feet, and there is even some evidence to support its use in treating hidradenitis suppurativa. Alitretinoin, meanwhile, is only really useful for hand dermatitis.

Retinoids do not affect your immune system, so there is no increased risk of infections. They can affect your liver and the fat levels in your blood, however, so these will both need to be monitored. All retinoids can also have severe effects during pregnancy, and are absolutely not to be used by people who are either pregnant or trying for a baby. Acitretin should not be used by younger women in particular, because it can stay in your system for up to 3 years; alitretinoin does not stay in your body for quite as long though, so girls could consider using this in certain circumstances.

Biological medicines: 'biologics'

There are now some newly designed injectable drugs, licensed and used for certain patients with severe forms of skin conditions like psoriasis, eczema, and hidradenitis suppurativa. These are referred to as biological medicines, or sometimes just 'biologics'.

A 'biologic' is a medication produced by living organisms, or at least by part of a living organism. They might be derived from humans, animals, or micro-organisms (including viruses or bacteria), in laboratories that use biotechnology. They are designed based on our knowledge of the diseases we want to treat, and target the specific responses in the body that are affected by each disease. Vaccines, anticancer drugs, and anti-inflammatory medications can all be produced this way; the anti-inflammatory versions we use in dermatology, for example, can then alter the pathways in our immune system that cause inflammation, which helps the skin as a result.

Most biologics need to be injected, and the other downside is that they cost a lot at the moment. They are therefore saved for people who don't respond to other treatments, because patients with severe forms of certain conditions have improved dramatically with biologics when other medications have failed. The other issue is that patients need to be regularly reviewed or tested for certain infections, because dampening down the immune system can make people more likely to get infected. It's also a chance to keep an eye out for any other possible problems, because most biologics are pretty new and data is still constantly being collected.

There are many biologics currently licensed in children and adolescents. This is changing all the time as new medicines are developed.

JAK inhibitors

JAK inhibitors are an emerging group of medications that may soon prove to be useful in treating hair and skin conditions. JAK is short for janus kinase, a molecule that plays a part in the way our immune systems function. Lots of the conditions mentioned in this book may be driven by abnormal activity in the immune system, and there is promising research that indicates JAK inhibitors are able to address this problem. Early results from trials treating atopic eczema, psoriasis, alopecia, and vitiligo look hopeful, although it may be some time before these kinds of treatments are licensed for use in the UK.

Miracle cures

You might see hundreds of adverts, read about amazing drugs in the media, or hear about other patients on internet forums that have had life-changing treatments. You may wonder why you are not being offered some of these.

Firstly, be careful about what you believe, and check where the information is coming from. Secondly, remember that there needs to be time to check that new drugs—especially ones that people will use long term—are safe and effective. Finally, keep expectations realistic. Even medicines that promise 'clear skin' do not always deliver this. The effects of many of these medications do not last for ever, and can stop working so well after being used for a long period of time. Alternatives may need to be considered, and there are studies on-going that are attempting to work out the best order to try things in. More personalized tests may be available in the future, which can tell an individual which medicine is likely to work best for them, but for now your doctor will offer you what they think is most appropriate.

There are strict criteria in the UK that guide what doctors can prescribe when, but if you really feel something isn't right for you then do discuss this with them; they should always be willing to listen and consider alternative options.

Resources

British Association of Dermatology information on systemic medications:
    https://www.skinhealthinfo.org.uk/a-z-conditions-treatments/

9

Sweating

 Key points

◆ Sweating is both a normal and important thing that our body does.

◆ Hyperhidrosis means sweating unusual amounts; it can affect any area of the body, but is most common on the palms, armpits, face, and scalp.

◆ There are various treatments that can help manage hyperhidrosis.

What is hyperhidrosis?

Hyperhidrosis is just a fancy word for extra sweating or perspiration. We all sweat to some degree—unless we have hypohidrosis, the opposite condition in which little-to-no sweat is produced—but when it happens too much, or in the wrong place and at the wrong time, then it can become a problem.

Sweat is produced by glands in the skin called eccrine glands, with the aim of keeping us cool when we get too hot or have started to exercise. For people with hyperhidrosis, however, an inappropriate amount of sweat can be produced, often at times when it's not necessary. This can happen in various different body parts, and the issues it causes therefore vary. Having very sweaty hands might make it difficult to write, or nerve-wracking to shake hands with people, whereas lots of sweat on clothing can affect a person's confidence and the clothes they choose to wear. Either way, this can have a huge impact on the way people feel and behave.

Eccrine glands

Eccrine glands—sometimes just called sweat glands—open directly onto the skin (Fig. 9.1) producing a thin, watery liquid. This contains a mixture of water and electrolytes, the small molecules such as sodium and chloride that give sweat its salty taste.

Skin Conditions in Young People. Tess McPherson, Oxford University Press. © Oxford University Press 2021.
DOI: 10.1093/oso/9780192895424.003.0009

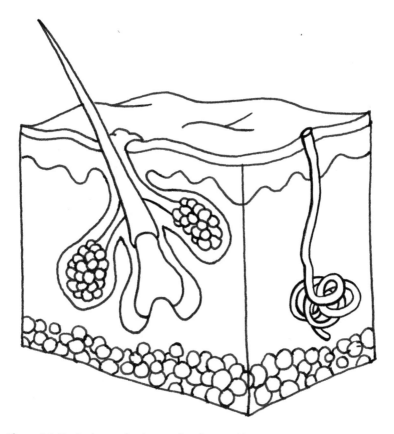

Figure 9.1 Eccrine/sweat gland opens directly onto skin.
© Reproduced courtesy of Damian Hale.

It's usually released in response to increasing temperatures and so we sweat when we are hot, but there are also other triggers that can induce sweating. Certain nerves can cause sweat to be released when we get nervous or embarrassed, for example, even if we're not that warm at the time.

Why do we sweat?

Mammals are the only animals that have developed the ability to sweat; we all do it, but humans, horses, and monkeys are some of the sweatiest. It's a pretty

69

effective way for us to cool ourselves down, as the sweat on our skin evaporates off and allows us to lose heat in the process. People who have conditions that mean they don't sweat quite as well can therefore get dangerously overheated.

Sweat also has a role in protecting the skin. It contains tiny little things known as antibodies, which the body produces to help fight infection.

Why do people get hyperhidrosis and what can you do?

Hyperhidrosis tends to be divided into two types:

1. Localized—affects a specific area
2. Generalized—affects the whole body, and may be caused by another underlying condition

The most common type of hyperhidrosis is the localized form; it often starts in adolescence, and does seem to be inherited. It might start in response to normal triggers, such as being a bit too hot, but these can then become abnormal. Stress, nerves, or excitement might set things off, and if the sweating then makes you feel more nervous it can become even more difficult to stop.

The sweatiest areas are usually the hands, feet, armpits, groin, face, and head, as these are the places we have the highest number of active sweat glands (Fig. 9.2). If you are overweight then losing a bit of weight can help, regardless of where you are feeling most sweaty; further treatments might differ slightly however, depending on which area is worst affected. Possible options include topicals (applied to the skin), tablets, and even something called iontophoresis (see next).

Treatments available for hyperhidrosis

Topical treatments

Topical antiperspirant treatments come in a variety of different forms, including roll-ons, wipes, creams, and gels, but all of them will usually contain the active ingredients aluminium chloride and glycopyrrolate. Antiperspirants aim to reduce sweating, whereas deodorants are designed to reduce smell (odour). Some products may even contain both. Antiperspirants are available over the counter or via the internet and come in different forms including wipes and gels.

All topical treatments that prevent sweating are likely to cause skin irritation when applied to wet skin, and so it is important to use them on completely dry

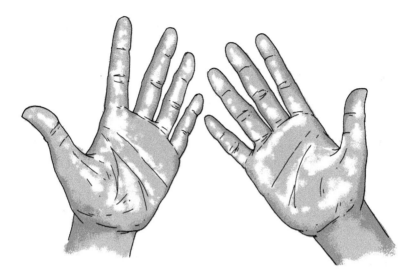

Figure 9.2 Sweaty palms.
© Reproduced courtesy of Damian Hale.

skin. The best way to do this is to wash your skin in the evening, dry it with a towel, or even a hair dryer on cold setting, then apply whatever cream or gel you have chosen. If your skin does become dry or sore, you might need to use a steroid ointment to treat the irritation; this way you can reduce the side effects while still making sure you get the benefits of the treatment.

Oral treatments

Tablets can be useful if sweating is more generalized, or if you're worried it might happen before a particular event. Most of the tablets are a type of medication called an anticholinergic. Anticholinergics are used for other conditions, including bed-wetting and irritable bowel syndrome, but can be helpful in stopping excessive sweating too. Your doctor will prescribe them to take either regularly or as needed, but it's worth having a trial run beforehand if you're using them for an important event. They can cause side effects such as dry eyes or dry mouth, so it's probably best to figure out what dose works for you ahead of time.

Iontophoresis

Iontophoresis is a process that involves running electrical currents through your skin, in order to then reduce how active the sweat glands are. You hire or buy a machine that passes a mild current through a small amount of water, then put your hands in the water while it is running. It does sound peculiar, but can be very useful for some people—especially those with sweaty hands.

Botox

Botox are the injections famous for treating wrinkles. They contain a form of toxin that can paralyse nerves, which is why people who have had Botox can't move their foreheads! This can be very effective for certain types of hyperhidrosis, particularly in the armpits, but the effect wears off quite quickly. The injections therefore need to be repeated fairly regularly, and as they aren't available on the NHS, this means sadly they might not be an option for everyone.

Remember: a bit of sweating is normal, but being drenched in sweat and leaving puddles is not. If you're worried or frustrated then speak to your doctor, or have a look at the links at the end of this chapter.

Resources

Patient support and useful tips and resources:

https://hyperhidrosisuk.org/

British Association of Dermatology information:

https://www.skinhealthinfo.org.uk/condition/hyperhidrosis/

10

Hair and hair loss (alopecia)

 Key points

- It's normal for hair and 'hairiness' to vary between people.

- Excessive body hair in areas where there is usually none—or at least very little—is known as hirsutism.

- Hair loss is called alopecia; it's very common, and there are many different causes

- The most common form of hair loss is androgenetic alopecia, better known as male-pattern baldness. In young people however, it's more likely to be an autoimmune condition called alopecia areata.

- Hair loss in alopecia areata can be anything from patchy to widespread. It might get better—although some young people have repeated episodes—and only rarely can lead to complete hair loss.

- Currently there are no totally safe or effective medications licensed for alopecia areata.

Normal hair

One of the big things that sets mammals apart from the rest of the animal kingdom is the fact that we have hair. There's still lots of variation between species, however, and it goes without saying that human hair grows in a different pattern to the hair we see on other animals. Hair in humans is present all over the body, aside from on the palms of the hands, the lips, and the genitals, and tends to be longest on the head. Exactly what it looks like will depend on so many things, including the genes you've inherited, your skin colour, and your age.

The only bit of hair that is 'living' sits in the hair follicle found within the skin. The visible bit of hair that comes out of the follicle—called the hair shaft—has

Skin Conditions in Young People. Tess McPherson, Oxford University Press. © Oxford University Press 2021.
DOI: 10.1093/oso/9780192895424.003.0010

no biochemical activity, and is not a living part of you. Each hair follicle will go through a stage of growth, after which the entire hair falls out; a new hair will then start to grow, beginning the cycle all over again. The hair follicles on your head all tend to be at different stages in this cycle, so it's normal to be continuously losing a few hairs. In fact, most people lose between 50 and 100 strands of hair per day.

Why do we have hair?

We don't totally understand the reasons that mammals have hair, but one thing we do know is that hair is important for temperature control. The hair on our head helps us with insulation, for example, by stopping us from losing body heat in the cold. Similarly, tiny muscles in your skin can make your hairs stand upright when it's cold. Better known as getting 'goosebumps', this helps to trap heat near the skin to keep warm. It's just as useful to have hair in sunnier weather as well, because the hair on your head will protect your scalp from sunburn. Plus, if you start getting a bit sweaty, the sweat can evaporate off your hair and cool you down in the process.

Pubic hair is a slightly different type of hair to the stuff on the rest of your body, but again we're not entirely sure what it's needed for. It's thought that it might help with cleanliness and protect against infections, although this is still debated.

Social aspects of hair

The role of hair has evolved significantly over the years, and it now does a lot more than just keep us warm. We style it, we cover it, we remove it; all of this means that it plays a big part in the way we're seen in society, and you could argue that this function of hair is just as important. It can define social groups—punks and skinheads of the 1970s, for example—as well as represent cultures, reflect genders, and shape identities. In the UK alone there have been massive changes over the past few centuries, in the length of hair, the colour of it, and the styles and the wigs you can choose from.

Removal of hair is also a very 'human' trait, and it's not a new thing; Ancient Egyptian women used to regularly remove both their pubic hair and head hair. It probably only became popular in the UK around the late 1800s, however, when Charles Darwin published his theory that we evolved from apes. This meant humans—particularly women—saw themselves as less ape-like, and therefore more sophisticated, if their bodies were hairless. Things only accelerated as fashionable clothing became more revealing, with the first bikini eventually leading to the first bikini wax in the 1980s. Male hair removal has also become increasingly popular, to the point that the beauty industry now markets both male and female grooming regimes.

There are no particular health benefits to removing bodily hair or pubic hair for most people. If you have hidradenitis suppurativa then it might be helpful (Chapter 7); otherwise, it's up to you. Hair removal can be achieved with a variety of techniques, including shaving, waxing, or laser, but none of these are routinely available on the NHS. Some of these—shaving in particular—can irritate eczema-prone skin and be associated with hair follicle infections, giving you spots that look a bit like acne. It is clearly a personal preference, but sometimes it's worth considering why we do this stuff?

Hirsutism

Hirsutism refers to excess hair on the body, in areas where there is normally little or none. Remember it's normal to have hair on most of our body, to some degree at least, and only very occasionally is excessive hair a sign of a serious medical condition.

In people born biologically female, or those who have transitioned to become female, hirsutism may be caused by an increase in—or increased sensitivity to—certain hormones. The most common condition in which this happens is polycystic ovarian syndrome (PCOS). In this case, hormonal treatments like the oral contraceptive pill can be really helpful; they will hopefully reduce hirsutism, as well as managing associated problems like acne (Chapter 3).

Even without any hormonal imbalance, people might consider their hair to be excessive and want to get rid of it. The methods available, such as waxing, shaving, bleaching and laser treatments, are all mentioned earlier, so it's just a case of working out what's best for you.

Alopecia

Alopecia is the opposite of hirsutism; it's the absence of hair from places it would normally grow. It can occur anywhere on the body, but tends to be most noticeable on the head. There are lots of different types of alopecia, from those that cause small amounts of hair loss to those that affect wide areas. This may either be scarring hair loss—when the hair follicle is damaged and hair cannot grow back—or non-scarring hair loss, where the hair follicle remains healthy and able to grow in the future.

Why me?—What can cause alopecia?

There are many different causes of hair loss, and most are pretty uncommon in young people. They would generally need a specialist doctor to diagnose them.

Causes of alopecia in young people include:

◆ **Inherited**—there are some genetic conditions that can affect the skin, hair, and sometimes the teeth and nails.

◆ **Underlying health conditions**—thyroid disease and anaemia—often caused by low iron in the blood—can both lead to generalized loss of hair, so treating the underlying health condition will help if this is the case.

◆ **Medicines**—certain drugs—particularly those used for chemotherapy—are designed to target fast-growing cancer cells. Hair cells grow quite quickly and are therefore also affected, but the hair will usually grow back once treatment is finished.

◆ **Telogen effluvium**—as we mentioned before, the hairs on our scalp are normally all at different stages of their growth cycle at any one time. A significant illness or pregnancy can push all the hair to cycle at once however, meaning they all fall out at the same time a few months later. This leads to a period of hair thinning, but should then settle over time.

◆ **Traction and rubbing**—hair styling techniques that pull hard on the hair, or put strain on the hair through use of heat treatments, can sometimes lead to hair loss. Rubbing over time will also do this; it's the reason we have less hair around the top of our socks, and explains why cats have less hair under their collars.

◆ **Trichotillomania**—persistent rubbing or pulling on hair is a condition called trichotillomania. It can be a serious problem, and is considered to be an obsessive-compulsive disorder that requires psychological support (see Chapter 16).

◆ **Infection**—fungal infection of the scalp can cause inflammation and hair loss, which can be treated with antifungal medications.

◆ **Inflammatory conditions**—uncommon inflammatory conditions, such as lupus and lichen planus, can also cause inflammation in the skin on the scalp. There are treatments available, but sometimes the hair loss caused by the inflammation is unfortunately scarring and therefore permanent.

◆ **Hormonal conditions**—a hormonal condition called androgenetic alopecia can cause hairs to become smaller, and is the reason males become bald as they get older. It may happen occasionally in people's teens and twenties however, and can also occur in females. Treatments aren't brilliant, but hormone tablets and a foam called minoxidil can sometimes help.

♦ **Autoimmune conditions**—the most common type of hair loss in young people is caused by an autoimmune condition called alopecia areata (see next).

What is alopecia areata?

Alopecia areata is a condition that causes non-scarring hair loss. It might just be patchy loss of head hair or facial hair (Fig. 10.1), but it can cover a

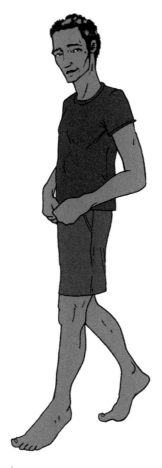

Figure 10.1 Patchy alopecia areata.
© Reproduced courtesy of Damian Hale.

wider spectrum; loss of all of the head hair—plus sometimes the eyebrows and eyelashes—is known as alopecia totalis, whereas if all body hair is lost, we call this alopecia universalis.

Patchy loss is the most common, and usually appears as well-defined, circular bald patches with normal healthy skin underneath. As there is no scarring and the follicles remain healthy, the hair is able to regrow. This is more likely to happen if only a small patch is affected, but the longer it goes without re-growing, the less chance there is of it coming back. Frustratingly this is really difficult to predict, and some people have patches that come and go for years.

Why me?—Why have I got alopecia areata?

Alopecia areata is an autoimmune condition. This kind of condition develops when your immune system, which is supposed to attack infections that might be harmful to your body, has ended up targeting bits of yourself instead. In alopecia areata, the hair follicles are the targets; how or why this happens isn't really understood though. What we do know is that it's more common in people who have—or have family members with—other conditions: asthma, eczema, or other autoimmune conditions such as type 1 diabetes, rheumatoid arthritis, vitiligo, or coeliac disease.

Most young people with alopecia areata are otherwise very healthy, with no significant medical conditions. It's unclear what triggers their immune systems to start attacking their hair follicles, although many patients have their own theories. Some identify a stressful event that happened just before the hair loss started for example, although stress is not clearly linked to alopecia. What's important to remember is that you haven't done anything wrong to cause your alopecia, and it's not contagious; you haven't caught it from somebody, and you can't give it to other people.

Management of alopecia

For most forms of alopecia, there is sadly no brilliant treatment or cure. Depending on the type you have, your doctor can discuss whether there are any treatments worth trying—just be careful with the ones that claim to work miracles!

Treatments for alopecia areata

A few patches of hair loss are very likely to grow back without any treatment, and so doing nothing may be just as good as anything else. As alopecia areata doesn't really cause your skin to become itchy and inflamed, and it's not going to make you feel unwell, long-term treatments need to be carefully considered; particularly if there are possible side effects that could impact on your health.

The most common treatment is a strong steroid ointment or scalp lotion, applied just to the areas affected. We can sometimes inject the steroid into the skin around problem areas as well, to treat the eyebrows, for example.

There are also tablet treatments available to suppress the immune system, stopping it from mistakenly attacking hair follicles. A steroid tablet called prednisolone can be given for a short time, as can the medication methotrexate (Chapter 8). Newer treatments known as janus kinase (JAK) inhibitors have also produced some promising hair growth in alopecia areata patients; they aren't yet licensed however, and we still don't really know about their long-term side effects.

The other issue is that, although we can suppress the immune system for a short time to allow hair to regrow, this probably won't change what happens over a longer period. Often when the tablets are stopped, hair falls out again and people feel even worse than before. In our experience, people who have tried a short course of tablets rarely want to do it again; with support, however, they end up able to be who they want to be, with hair or without it.

How to manage having alopecia?

Losing your hair can have a massive impact on how you feel about yourself, especially if this happens in your teens and twenties. The key is to have realistic expectations, and understand what can and can't be done. The uncertainty of whether your hair will grow back or not is understandably difficult to deal with, but unfortunately there's no easy way to predict what's going to happen.

Thankfully there's lots that can be done to help you manage in the meantime. Particular hairstyles, cosmetic products, wigs, hairpieces, hats, and scarves; these can all be useful in covering bald patches. Boys are often keen to just shave their head at a fairly early stage rather than wear a wig, but obviously it varies from person to person. Don't be embarrassed to ask a hairdresser for advice, as it's likely you won't be the first person they've seen with alopecia.

Alternatively, you may choose to leave alopecia uncovered. This is a very personal thing, and will probably depend on where and to what extent you have lost hair. Widespread alopecia can cause a huge sense of loss initially, and can be really difficult to cope with when it first happens. Some people still find it easier to leave it as it is however, or to think about positive options such as wigs, hairpieces, and tattoos.

There is evidence that the stigma attached to hair loss has reduced over time, which can only be a good thing. Charities like Alopecia UK have been really important in this, as have celebrities and other positive role models who post about it online. That's not to say it makes things easy; just that increased awareness means young people might find it possible to make alopecia a positive part of their identity. Older patients would rarely ever let anyone see their head exposed, for example, but this is certainly not the case now. Young people with alopecia are starting to appreciate that the skin doesn't hurt or itch, that it doesn't make you unhealthy, and that bald can definitely be beautiful (Fig. 10.2).

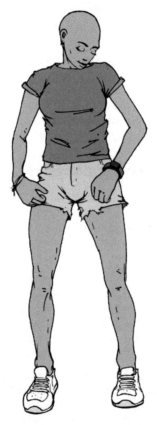

Figure 10.2 Some young people choose not to cover their alopecia—it is a personal choice.

© Reproduced courtesy of Damian Hale.

Dealing with other people

A commonly occurring problem involves other people thinking your hair loss is because of cancer treatment, which can feel awkward and uncomfortable. Often, it's just because they are concerned about your health, so it's probably easiest to discuss things openly. It won't stop you from having friends or relationships, because people worth bothering with won't judge anyone on their lack of hair—no matter what the reason is.

Another issue we sometimes see is that the parents or carers of young people with alopecia really struggle, and—in some cases—push for aggressive and potentially unsafe treatments. In these situations, it can be the young people themselves who have to reassure their parents and family that they are OK. It shouldn't really be the role of someone with alopecia to reassure others, but I am constantly impressed by the strength of young people who do this. If other people can support and accept you as you are, however, that works out better for everybody.

Last thoughts

Hair is funny stuff, and we don't know really why we have it in the ways we do. It certainly plays an important role in how we present ourselves; you just have to look at all the money people spend on hairdressers and hair removal to see that. It definitely isn't the be-all and end-all though, and hair should therefore not be allowed to affect who and how we are.

Resources

Young people's experiences of hair loss:
> http://healthtalk.org/young-peoples-experiences/alopecia/topics

Alopecia support for patients of all ages:
> https://www.alopecia.org.uk/advice-for-children-and-young-people-with-alopecia

11

Skin pigmentation and vitiligo

 Key points

- The colour of your skin is controlled by something called pigment; the amount of pigment in your skin could be increased—or decreased—for a number of reasons.

- Inflammation can 'stain' the skin, because it changes the amount of pigment produced by the skin in that area.

- Vitiligo is a common autoimmune condition, which causes pigment to be lost from some areas of skin.

Skin colour

Your skin colour is decided by a blend of coloured substances in the skin: a palate of red, blue, orange, and brown. The main colour—also referred to as pigment—is a brown substance called melanin, made by the skin cells known as melanocytes. How light or dark your skin colour is therefore depends on how many melanocytes you have, as well as how they are working. Higher levels of melanin in the skin make it darker and less prone to sun damage for example, whereas lighter skin—containing less melanin—might burn more easily.

Thanks to melanin, humans have developed an amazing and unique range of skin colours. Our skins have adapted to a variety of different living environments over time, finding levels of melanin that suit environments that are either sunny, cold, or in between. Variations in skin colour—or even just patches of pigment change—can unfortunately be used as a cause of division between humans however, or a reason for stigmatization. Clearly this needs to change. People are hopefully now aware that skin colour is no basis, ever, for how people should be viewed or treated.

Skin Conditions in Young People. Tess McPherson, Oxford University Press. © Oxford University Press 2021. DOI: 10.1093/oso/9780192895424.003.0011

Increased skin pigment changes

Whatever colour your skin, there are various ways in which its pigment might be altered. Moles and freckles are one of the most common examples of local areas of increased skin pigment, which you can either be born with or later develop. They are essentially just collections of melanocytes, and the number of melanocytes there will dictate how dark the freckles and moles are.

Some people find their freckles only 'come out' when they've been in the sun for a while. The reason this happens—and the reason that your skin gets darker in the sun in general—is that melanocytes produce a brown pigment called melanin in response to sunlight, which protects your skin from burning. A suntan may then appear as a result. Although tanning is better for your skin than sunburn, it can still lead to sun damage and skin cancer if you overdo it; that's why the pigment in fake tan is probably safer!

Decreased skin pigment changes

The amount of pigment in the skin can also be reduced for a number of reasons. Just as you can be born with dark moles or freckles, you might have paler, less pigmented areas that have been there since you were a baby. Loss of pigment might even be widespread rather than patchy; a condition called albinism can cause generalized pigment changes that are present from birth, resulting in skin that is vulnerable to sun damage.

Even if no pigment changes are present when you are born, scars can appear throughout your life—after a deep cut for example—and may leave pale patches of skin that end up being permanent.

Certain infections may also cause pigment loss, although some are more common than others. Pityriasis versicolor is probably the best example, a yeast infection often seen in young people that causes pale spotty areas on the back. There are several other causes, all of which are rare and unusual, but if you're worried or unsure about anything then it's probably best to get your doctor to have a look.

Inflammation and pigment changes

One of the most common causes of a change in pigment, and therefore skin colour, is inflammation. Inflammation in the skin—eczema, psoriasis, or any rash really—can upset the melanocytes and cause them to produce more or less pigment. The exact changes will depend on your skin type, as well as the cause of the inflammation. For instance, psoriasis often causes paler areas, whereas a rash called lichen planus causes an increase in pigment; eczema, on the other hand, can cause either. Post-inflammatory pigment change can be particularly noticeable in darker skin types. People often worry that it's due steroid use, but it's not; it's the inflammation that affects the pigment. It is not 'scarring' and will generally settle over time. It can take a long time—months, or even years—but moisturizers and good skin control will always help.

Vitiligo is another condition that commonly causes pigment changes, and in some patients, it can be really difficult to tell this apart from the post-inflammatory loss of pigment described earlier. Both are acquired, by which we mean they appear sometime after birth, and the fact that there isn't always a clear period of inflammation before skin turns pale can make things even trickier. The easiest way to tell the difference is that vitiligo tends to occur in distinct blocks of skin, which have no pigment whatsoever; inflammation, on the other hand, just causes skin to become slightly paler, in areas that are less well defined.

It might not seem that important, but getting the right diagnosis is really helpful when it comes to working out how to manage things.

What is vitiligo?

Vitiligo is 'an acquired chronic depigmentation disorder, which results in a loss of functional melanocytes'. That all sounds very scientific, but if we break the definition down it's just saying that:

◆ **Acquired**—you aren't born with it, but it appears at some point during your life

◆ **Chronic**—it happens over a long period of time

◆ **Depigmentation**—your skin loses its pigment, and therefore its colour

◆ **Loss of functional melanocytes**—and this happens because not enough of the skin cells that produce pigment are working properly

The end result is that areas of skin lose their natural pigment and colour, and so they start to turn white. If you have pale skin it therefore won't be as obvious—especially if you have no suntan—but if you have dark skin it can be very noticeable from the beginning.

Vitiligo is pretty common. Around 1% of the world's population has it, and in countries like India the number can be as high as 8%. It affects both men and women equally, and about half of the patients with vitiligo will have developed it before they turn 20.

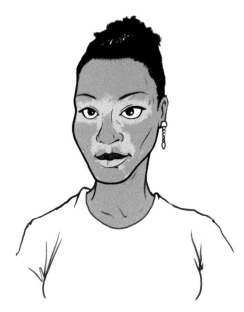

Figure 11.1 Vitiligo.
© Reproduced courtesy of Damian Hale.

The most common form of vitiligo is called *non-segmental vitiligo*. Most often this affects the face—particularly around the eyes—the hands, feet, genitals, and sometimes the elbows and knees. It's usually symmetrical, affecting both sides of the body at once, and can either appear in small patches or be more widespread (Fig. 11.1). The speed at which it develops may also vary, with the number of new patches sometimes increasing quite fast in certain people.

Why me?—Why have I got vitiligo?

It's important to know that you've done nothing to cause your vitiligo, because—although it's not entirely clear why melanocytes stop functioning in certain areas of patients' skin—it's certainly not the fault of the patient.

We think the immune system could be involved, as vitiligo is linked to other autoimmune conditions. These kinds of conditions develop when your immune system—which is supposed to attack any infections that might be harmful to your body—has ended up targeting bits of you instead. In vitiligo it's the melanocytes that are the targets, and so they stop being able to make pigment for the skin as a result.

If you have a family member with another autoimmune condition, including vitiligo, then there's a higher chance you may develop vitiligo yourself. It's not all genetic, however; there are cases of identical twins—who have the same genes—where one twin develops vitiligo and the other doesn't. This indicates there must be other triggers involved, and these may include chemical exposure, injury, or friction to the skin. Many people may also feel that stress, or stressful events, have played a role, although the evidence for this is limited. As discussed through this book, it is important not to feel that your 'stress' is responsible; there are ways to address how stressed you feel (Chapter 17), and blaming yourself for your skin condition is never necessary.

Thyroid disease is the autoimmune condition most commonly linked to vitiligo, and up to half of adults with vitiligo will have a problem with their thyroid too. The thyroid is an organ in your neck that helps manage your metabolism, and so it's important to keep an eye on your weight and your energy levels and consult your doctor if you're worried about thyroid problems. Thankfully, however, many young people with vitiligo have no other health issues, and may even be protected from certain conditions. It seems that people with vitiligo have a lower risk of a type of skin cancer called melanoma, although it's not entirely clear why; it might simply be that they're just better at protecting their skin from sunburn.

Impact of having vitiligo

Even though vitiligo isn't generally itchy, sore, or infectious, it can still have a huge impact on people's lives. A major problem for some people with vitiligo is the way it looks, and the fact that this can affect the way they're viewed by both themselves and others.

Patients with vitiligo do report prejudice, and sometimes even clear discrimination. This can be worse in certain cultures or countries than others. In India, for example, people with vitiligo have been avoided in the past, because leprosy—an infectious disease that can also cause pale skin, and which is often mistaken for vitiligo—is also more common in that part of the world.

Learning to deal with staring and comments can be emotionally demanding, but there's hope that this is getting easier as people become more informed. There are now supermodels with vitiligo, and even a Barbie doll with the condition. While that doesn't necessarily make everything magically better, it should at least mean that more people know what vitiligo is, and hopefully cut down on the number of insensitive questions patients with vitiligo have to deal with from others too.

What can I do?

Firstly, make sure your diagnosis is correct. People can be told they have vitiligo even though the pale areas on their skin are caused by something else, so if you're not sure, then get a doctor to take a look. They may want advice from a dermatologist in order to be certain.

The most important thing to then do—if you do have vitiligo—is to protect your skin. Patches of vitiligo on the skin can be easily sunburnt, and so sun protection is key. This will also help if the appearance of your skin is a big worry, as stopping the surrounding skin from getting tanned will keep the affected areas less obvious. Don't overdo it however, because we need sunlight on our skin to produce vitamin D; it may therefore be worth taking vitamin D supplements if you're reducing your sun exposure significantly.

Avoiding tight clothing may be advised, but this is not always practical. Instead, using moisturizers and emollients can make your skin feel good, and will possibly reduce rubbing and friction from your clothing too. It's thought that this rubbing can contribute to vitiligo in some areas, and so you might find this helps slightly. There are also certain chemicals that have been observed to trigger vitiligo, including some hair dyes, deodorants or perfumes, cosmetics, and rubber gloves. This usually happens when they've been used for a long time—at work, for example—but if you suspect this could be the cause, it may be worth avoiding these chemicals too.

On top of all this there are treatments for vitiligo that act to slow its progress, and even give you back some pigment. At the moment, however, you cannot cure it completely; no treatment has been shown to return your natural skin colour entirely, and the vitiligo often reappears regardless.

Active treatments

Whether or not your vitiligo resolves on its own, or even whether it responds to treatment, will depend on a variety of factors. Treatments for vitiligo do seem to work better in certain situations; newer areas appear to be more treatable, and younger people respond better than adults on the whole.

Treating the face: Certain areas—particularly the face—seem to be more likely to resolve on their own, and also tend to respond better to treatment. Areas that have been present for months to years are less likely to be treatable, however, and may not regain their pigment.

Treating the hands and feet: The hands and feet often won't regain their pigment, even if they are treated. It may be that you decide not to try and treat these areas, but use clothing or cover-up products instead.

Treating the genital area: Many vitiligo patients have patches that affect their genital area. This can cause embarrassment, and stop people from dating or having sex. Unfortunately, the genital area is difficult to treat, because the skin there is very delicate. The best way to manage this might therefore be to try being open and honest with your partner, when the time is right. Intimate relationships are most rewarding when based on mutual respect, and not on body shaming of any kind. You could always choose to use cover-up products on the area, but really, it's whatever you feel comfortable with; we'd still just recommend talking to a healthcare professional if vitiligo is causing you problems here.

There are a few different options in terms of medication for vitiligo. Anti-inflammatory treatments, like those used in skin conditions such as eczema (Chapter 4), can reduce the number of immune cells that are hanging around and targeting melanocytes. Strong corticosteroid creams are examples that have been shown to work for vitiligo, as has an ointment known as tacrolimus.

Tacrolimus is a non-steroidal anti-inflammatory treatment; it's usually recommended as the first choice, ahead of the corticosteroid creams. This is because the use of strong steroid creams to treat vitiligo—particularly on the face, or on larger areas of skin—is less safe than it is in eczema. It also may be less effective, and given that there are risks with overuse, tacrolimus is often the preferred option. The tablet versions of steroids can also give a short-term increase in pigment but, as with the creams, the side effects need to be considered (Chapter 8); especially as they won't 'cure' vitiligo long term.

In certain cases, special light treatments can be prescribed and given in the hospital. This might seem strange, because the advice is generally to avoid the sun if you've got vitiligo. It can reduce the immune response, however, which may help increase the levels of pigment for people with certain skin types. This has to be carefully thought through though, particularly in young people.

Aside from this, there is sadly not much else available at the moment. Some people have looked into certain dietary supplements, but only in small trials, and so there's not yet any strong evidence that changing your diet will improve your vitiligo. There are plenty of other treatments being trialled currently too, and some of these are showing some potentially positive results. Be careful paying a lot for private treatments, or taking experimental drugs that aren't being used in clinical trials, however. You don't want to risk your health on treatments that might not actually be safe.

With any treatment, it's always necessary to think about how likely it is to help; weighing up the possible side effects or risks is important too. It may be good to try for a bit—focusing on new areas perhaps—but if nothing is happening, then it's not worth pushing on. Some people, on the other hand, decide not to try active treatments at all, and that is also totally fine.

Cover up areas

Some people decide that they want to cover their areas of vitiligo. You can use fake tan or tinted moisturizer, and there are special camouflage creams that can do this too. These can completely match your normal skin pigment, and the fact that they're waterproof means they can safely be used for sport and swimming. There's waterproof mascara or eyelash dye if your eyelashes are affected, although lots of patients learn to love their pale eyelashes. People often find that the creams work best on smaller areas, or on the face rather than other parts of the body. You might use them just for certain occasions, or instead not use them at all. Whatever you decide is absolutely fine.

Accepting that your skin is different and just getting on with things won't always feel easy, but it's often the most helpful way to live. If it's making you feel bad, or if people are being unkind, then it's really important to talk to someone who can help, however. Just remember that vitiligo should not stop you doing anything you want to, or prevent you from being whoever you want to be.

'Own your vitiligo, don't let your vitiligo own you' (vitiligosupport.org.uk)

Resources

Patient support charity with great resources. It also shares struggles and tips from other patients who have dealt with the condition:

http://www.vitiligosupport.org.uk/

Charity that offers free support for cosmetic camouflage:

https://www.changingfaces.org.uk/

British Association of Dermatology information:

https://www.britishskinfoundation.org.uk/vitiligo
https://www.skinhealthinfo.org.uk/condition/skin-camouflage/

12

Genital skin

 Key points

- Your genitals are as unique as you are, and there is no one specific way they should look or size that they should be.

- Sometimes the appearance of your genitals will vary, or they might seem to have additional marks on them. These are actually fairly common and therefore nothing to be overly concerned about.

- Some skin conditions can affect the genitals; there are treatments available for these, however, so you should seek medical advice if you're worried about anything.

- If you are sexually active, practice safe sex and take steps to ensure you don't become a parent sooner than you plan to. Get screened regularly for STIs. If you don't feel ready to talk to a partner about any of this, then—as a general rule of thumb—you're probably not ready to sleep with them either.

Normal stages of development

The changes you experience as you move from childhood into adolescence can seem a bit strange at times, but they are all entirely normal; it's essentially just your body transitioning from a child's into an adult's. Whether you're a boy or girl, you will probably grow taller, your skin will become greasier, and you may even notice your voice changing too.

You might undergo some other changes alongside all this, and these are the ones that people sometimes find a bit more embarrassing. Girls will have their first periods and start to develop breasts, as well as pubic and underarm hair. Boys also grow hair under their arms and around their genitals, and may notice that their genitals are getting bigger too. This tends to begin with the testicles

Skin Conditions in Young People. Tess McPherson, Oxford University Press. © Oxford University Press 2021.
DOI: 10.1093/oso/9780192895424.003.0012

and scrotum (or 'balls')—before the penis becomes longer and then eventually wider.

The rate at which all of this happens varies widely between individuals. This can be a bit annoying if you're one of the first—or last—among your friends to develop in these areas, especially because it can sometimes feel like it's really obvious. It's normal to feel self-conscious about it all, but just bear in mind that nearly all of your peer group will feel the same way; some just appear to hide it better!

These changes all happen in order to turn your body into one that is ready to reproduce. Basically, everything is getting itself ready to have kids, and it's possible for girls to fall pregnant as soon as they've had their first period. Just because you *can*, however, doesn't mean you should! If you're thinking about becoming sexually active then it's usually an idea to speak to somebody about contraception first, and either your GP or local sexual health clinic could be a good place to start. If you're not feeling ready for this yet then that's equally normal, so don't let yourself be pressured into anything too soon.

Variants of normal

Boys

The appearance of the penis varies widely between boys, and there is no one look that is 'normal' for everyone. There's also a significant difference between a non-erect penis and a fully erect one, so whether it seems 'big' or 'small' in the resting state is fairly irrelevant. The testicle and scrotum tend to vary in size too, and because one testicle is usually higher than the other, they can often be slightly asymmetrical.

You might not have much hair in this area at all, or alternatively it could grow all the way round from your bottom to your belly button. Either is entirely normal.

Pearly penile papules

These are small, skin-coloured bumps, generally arranged in one or more rows, and are located around the head of the penis. They are perfectly normal, and tend to get less noticeable with age.

Girls

The vulva is the part of the female genitalia that you can see, and consists of both outer and inner lips that are known as labia. Although this area is commonly referred to as the vagina, the vagina is actually just the tube connecting these outer parts to the uterus (or 'womb').

Contrary to what is often seen online—particularly on pornography sites—there isn't a single specific way that vulvas have to look in order to be 'normal'. The outer and inner lips of the vulva can vary considerably in size and length, and usually will become larger during puberty. Initially one might be slightly bigger than the other; sometimes this evens out, sometimes this little bit of asymmetry persists, but either is absolutely normal.

Vulval papillae

These are small 'growths' that sometimes occur in women, either on the inner lips of the vulva or at the opening of the vagina. They might look like small smooth bumps, or alternatively could be little 'finger-like' lumps, and usually grow in lines or patches. They're pretty harmless, and so don't need investigation or treatment.

Both

Fordyce spots

These are the small glands in the skin—known as sebaceous glands—that normally produce an oily kind of substance, and appear as tiny yellow or white 'spots'. They are located on the inside of the lips and cheeks, as well as on the genitals. Boys may find that they appear on the head and shaft of the penis, whereas in girls they may be seen on the vulva; either way they are totally harmless.

Angiokeratomas

These are fairly common marks that can be seen anywhere on the body, but are often found on the genitals; in this case they're called 'angiokeratoma of Fordyce'. They appear as red, purple, or sometimes black 'spots', and represent tiny blood vessels that have expanded near the surface of the skin. They aren't dangerous at all, and therefore are nothing to worry about.

Moles

You can get moles on any part of your skin, and that includes the skin on your genitals. They're not usually any more worrying than a mole elsewhere, but if they're new or changing you should still probably get them checked out by your doctor.

Skin conditions that can affect the genitals

We've talked a bit about what is 'normal' in terms of appearance, but it's also important to remember that your genital skin—like the skin on any other part of your body—should generally feel comfortable and free of symptoms too. Any discomfort in this area, including itching, soreness, a bad odour, or change in discharge, is not 'just normal' and therefore needs looking into. It could signal a minor infection, or instead a specific skin condition; even if it might be slightly embarrassing, it's best to tell either your GP or an adult you trust in order to get this sorted out.

Common skin conditions seen on other parts of the body can also affect your genitals—including psoriasis, eczema, hidradenitis suppurativa, and vitiligo (Chapters 6, 4, 7, and 11). Treatment for skin problems affecting genitals is similar to other, which is discussed in detail in earlier chapters. As it can look a bit different in this area however, and, given the understandable distress it can cause, it often needs stronger treatments prescribed by a skin expert in order to manage it quickly. Certain forms of eczema that develop specifically in the genitals can be very itchy, and if the affected skin becomes thicker due to rubbing or scratching this itching can get even worse. Often it will be noticed because you have eczema elsewhere, although in some cases it might only be seen in the genital area. Psoriasis is similar, in that it can affect the genitals despite not really being that obvious on the rest of the body; like eczema, if this is the only place it occurs then it could need a specialist to diagnose.

Rarely, conditions that affect other parts of the body may also cause skin changes, in which case genital skin can sometimes be involved. Inflammatory bowel diseases such as Crohn's are the most common example, affecting the bottom, groin, and potentially the vulva. This might be difficult to diagnose, especially if it happens in the absence of any bowel symptoms, and will need to be managed by both a skin and a bowel specialist.

Specific genital skin conditions

In addition to everything mentioned here, there are also a few skin conditions that tend to involve genital skin specifically. These need to be managed—at least at the start—by a dermatologist or gynaecologist with a specialist interest, as they can sometimes be missed or treated incorrectly.

These conditions can be seen in both girls and boys, although seem to be more common in girls.

Lichen sclerosus (LS)

LS is a condition that causes itching in the genital area, and scratching can sometimes lead to this skin becoming sore. Initially it is often mistaken for thrush, or sometimes even worms in younger girls. It won't settle without the correct diagnosis and treatment, however, and plenty of people use a lot of over-the-counter medications for thrush before somebody realizes why they aren't working.

LS makes the skin appear a bit dry, pale, and wrinkled, sometimes with some fairly striking purple bruises in the affected areas. This can affect the vulval skin in girls, or the skin around the head of the penis in boys. The area around the bottom known as perianal skin may also be involved. In rare cases there will be similar patches on the rest of the skin, which can mean they are a bit harder to treat.

We aren't yet completely sure why people get this condition, although there are lots of theories. It seems to be more common in girls, who tend to develop it either before puberty or after menopause. It also appears to be more likely in those with a family history of certain autoimmune conditions: thyroid disease, vitiligo, and lupus are all examples of these.

There's also a bit of uncertainty about how LS develops, although it's been suggested that the leaking of tiny drops of urine—often not even seen—could be a potential cause. In males this then leads to irritation of the head of the penis, as the urine is trapped there by the foreskin. Although it is possible that a similar thing could occur in girls and women, this is yet to be proven.

The usual treatment—in both boys and girls—is a strong steroid ointment applied to the affected areas. This needs to be done according to a specific regime, and patients are also advised to avoid soaps and shower gels as part of treatment. If left untreated then LS can sometimes lead to scarring, but if managed effectively it's generally easy to keep away. It may improve in some girls around puberty but it is not uncommon to get flare ups which need on-going management. This can be more common when on holiday, so always remember to pack your ointment when going away! If boys find that they are experiencing scarring despite treatment however, circumcision (removal of the foreskin) may be needed in order to properly treat the condition.

Lichen planus (LP)

This fairly rare condition is closely related to LS, although usually causes the genitals to be sore rather than itchy. Lichen planus can also affect other parts of the body, including the skin, scalp, nails, mouth, and bowels.

The genital subtype often needs to be managed in a specialist clinic, at least until it's under good control. It will initially be treated in a similar way to LS, but sometimes tablets may also be required.

Infections that can occur on the genitals (including sexually transmitted infections)

It's not within the scope of this book to give detailed information about all the possible infections that can affect the genitals. The best and most simple advice is that if you're sexually active, and you notice a new ulcer, sore, growth, or discharge, you should take yourself to your local sexual health clinic to get tested.

Some people can find talking about all this stuff slightly embarrassing, but these aren't things you should just live with. Whatever the skin condition, it's important that you get it seen by a doctor and are given the treatment you need.

Resources

Normal variation of penises:
> https://www.healthline.com/health/types-of-penises

Normal variations of vulvas:
> https://www.healthline.com/health/womens-health/lopsided-vagina

This should really be called great wall of vulvas!:
> http://www.greatwallofvagina.co.uk/home

British Association of Dermatology—lichen sclerosus information:
> https://www.skinhealthinfo.org.uk/condition/lichen-sclerosus-in-female-children/
> https://www.skinhealthinfo.org.uk/condition/lichen-sclerosus-in-males/

13

Moles and marks

➜ Key points

◆ Lots of different marks can appear on skin; they might either be present at birth, or acquired throughout life.

◆ Most of these are benign, which means they pose no threat to your health.

◆ Removing a mark for cosmetic reasons will always leave a scar, and it's hard to predict what that scar will look like.

What is a mole?

Naevus—or naevi, if there's more than one of them—is the medical term for a mole. It's usually used to refer to birthmarks, but many moles can develop after birth. They're extremely common, and most people have about 10 to 40 of them somewhere on their skin (Fig. 13.1).

Common naevi are harmless collections of dark-coloured skin cells, and typically appear as small brown, tan, or pink spots. You might be born with them, or alternatively you might develop them as you grow older.

The type you're born with are known as congenital moles. These vary in size, and can be very large in some people. Big congenital naevi are sometimes associated with other problems, and can put people who have them at increased risk of skin cancer; most, however, are totally harmless, and can be there for a lifetime without causing any issues.

Acquired moles, meanwhile, are extremely common. Most people develop some during childhood and adolescence, although we don't really know why. We do know that most are completely safe though, and it's extremely uncommon to have a cancerous mole before adulthood. Having said that, if you

Skin Conditions in Young People. Tess McPherson, Oxford University Press. © Oxford University Press 2021.
DOI: 10.1093/oso/9780192895424.003.0013

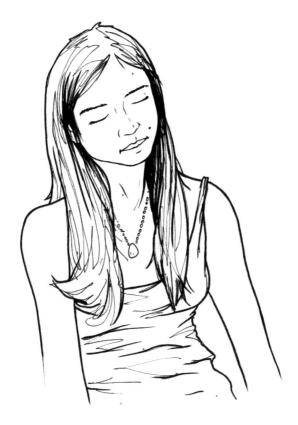

Figure 13.1 Moles are common—we pretty much all have them.
© Reproduced courtesy of Damian Hale.

have a mole which is getting bigger or looks very different, then it's still always worth getting it checked out.

Removing moles

It's rare for a young person to develop a dangerous mole; what's much more common is that they don't like the way a mole looks or feels. Attitudes vary massively between people, because while one person might just think of their mole as a beauty spot, another could feel like theirs is a huge problem.

We do see patients who get teased or bullied about their moles—particularly if they are on their faces—and it's important to take this seriously. On balance, if the mole is big or in the way then we can consider removing it, even if it might not be dangerous to leave it there. Young people can sometimes think their mole looks ugly despite the fact that nobody else notices it, however, or believe that if a certain mole was gone then everything would be OK. It's in these situations that we really have to consider whether removing the mole is the right thing to do.

Scars

One of the reasons we are cautious about removing moles is that we can't do it without leaving a scar. While you might be happy to accept a scar in order to get rid of a cancerous mark, getting rid of a benign, non-cancerous mole is a different story. People often feel that the scar would be less ugly than a mole, but that's not necessarily true.

Firstly, moles are not ugly; they are a normal part of us. Secondly—and this is something that not everyone is aware of—scars can be bumpy, lumpy, or itchy, and even form something called a keloid. A keloid occurs when the scar tissue becomes overgrown, producing a lump that can be much bigger than the original wound. It's most likely to happen on the head, neck, and upper chest, which are areas that people most often want moles removed from. **You know what your mole looks like, but by getting rid of it you're trading it in for an unpredictable scar**; some will heal well, but nobody can promise you that it will be perfect and neat.

We try to only make a scar if it is needed, and so benign moles aren't removed on the NHS for the reason that they don't usually need to be. Even if you are thinking about going privately to have a mole removed, make sure you get proper advice about the scar you could end up with and then consider things carefully. You might decide you're able to live with your mole; it's a part of you after all, and may not be as awful as it seems.

Vascular marks

Some common birth marks are caused by blood vessels in the skin, and so we call them vascular marks. One good example is a 'port wine stain', which starts off at birth as a flat red mark—often on the face—then over time can become more raised. Occasionally these vascular marks will be seen with other health issues that need managing, but it may be possible to treat the birthmark itself too. Laser treatments can shrink the blood vessels and make them less noticeable, although this won't get rid of the mark completely.

Cosmetic camouflage

Whatever the mark is on your skin, there are options if you feel uncomfortable leaving it exposed. The choices will depend on what and where it is, but flat marks in particular—for example, port wine stains or vitiligo—can be covered with special products that people find really helpful for some occasions.

It's important to stay realistic about these things, however; it might not be possible to get rid of a mole, or hide a mark entirely. Remember that they are more normal than you think, and if you can you should learn to love them!

Resources

NHS information on moles:

> https://www.nhs.uk/conditions/moles/

Charity that offers free advice and support for cosmetic camouflage for all skin conditions. Self-referral available through the website:

> https://www.changingfaces.org.uk

14

Skin infections and infestations

 Key points

- Healthy skin is covered in millions of different bugs, most of which are harmless.

- Sometimes bugs can cause problems, including flaky skin, itchy skin, hair loss, or even abscesses.

- Certain skin conditions can make you more likely to get infections.

- If your immune system is not working properly—for whatever reason—you are more susceptible to all types of infection, not just ones that affect the skin.

- It is important to diagnose skin infections correctly, so that you then get the right treatments.

Healthy bugs

Our skin is covered in loads of bugs. In fact, there are so many bacteria on our bodies that we are actually carrying around more bacterial DNA than our own, human DNA most of the time. Normal bugs on the skin aren't just bacteria, however; we have a mixture of bacteria, viruses, yeast, and fungi, that together make up our skin 'flora'.

This is sometimes referred to as the 'microbiome', a whole world that we are still finding out lots about. Most of this microbiome is healthy, and ideally made up of a wide variety of bugs. Loss of variety can cause problems; accumulation of a specific bacteria called *Staph aureus* in eczema can lead to flare ups, for example.

Skin Conditions in Young People. Tess McPherson, Oxford University Press. © Oxford University Press 2021.
DOI: 10.1093/oso/9780192895424.003.0014

We start picking up this variety of bugs from the moment we are born. All of us have some that could potentially cause problems, but as long as the immune system keeps them in check they don't cause noticeable issues. A fungus might sit on our skin without us realizing, as just another part of the microbiome; however, if it's not kept under control by the immune system and the balance gets upset, that's when it can lead to something like athlete's foot appearing. Infections or infestations can also be caused by unwelcome visitors from outside the microbiome—scabies and head lice are a couple of examples.

A clinical infection is one that causes a medical problem that needs treatment. Whether or not you develop one will depend on lots of things: the genes you've inherited, the type of skin you have, how well your immune system is working, and the kind of bugs you've been exposed to.

Problem bugs

There are certain bugs that more commonly cause infections in young people, and the most important ones to know about are covered next.

Viruses

Viruses are tiny 'infectious agents'. They cannot survive on their own, so instead they enter cells in the body and use them to make more virus, before then spreading these copies around.

Herpes simplex virus (HSV)

This is the virus that causes both cold sores and genital herpes. It is pretty common, and appears as small water-filled blisters—known as vesicles—that are often pretty sore.

Genital herpes is generally spread during sex, whereas cold sores caused by HSV are just passed around by close contact. The virus can sometimes hang around in your nerve cells, so tends to keep affecting the same area of skin supplied by that nerve; this is why some people are prone to getting repeated cold sores. They can be treated with antiviral medications, either in the form of a cream or tablet, whereas genital herpes can only really be treated by the tablet version.

HSV can also cause a severe, widespread rash in people with eczema, known as *eczema herpeticum* (Chapter 4).

Varicella zoster virus (VZV)

VZV is the virus that causes chickenpox. Like HSV, it can hide out in nerve cells and then reappear later as *shingles*.

Molluscum contagiosum

Molluscum are little bumps on the skin caused by a poxvirus. They are common in younger children, but can develop at any age. People respond differently to the molluscum infection; some will get just one spot and it will then clear quickly, whereas other people—including those with eczema—will have widespread spots that can take much longer to clear up.

Unfortunately, there's no brilliant treatment for molluscum, although lots have been tried. They should disappear over time, as long as you have a well-functioning immune system. If you have eczema around the molluscum this should be managed. They tend to get quite inflamed when your immune system starts to notice them, which can look quite dramatic; normally this doesn't mean you need medication, but instead that your molluscum are on their way out! Try not to squeeze them, as the spots are full of new copies of the virus that you might spread around. There is a small chance they can leave scars, so it's best to just leave them alone—it can take an annoyingly long time, but they will go eventually.

Human papilloma virus (HPV)

Warts are the rough 'hyperkeratotic' bumps—collections of cells in the skin producing too much keratin—caused by HPV. Warts seem to like the hands, feet, genitals, and face in particular. There are lots of different types of HPV, and some are more likely to cause skin warts than others.

Warts on the skin can be a pain. As with molluscum, there are no great treatments to cure warts; it's just a case of waiting for the immune system to deal with them. It can sometimes take years for your immune system to notice that they are there, and for people on treatments that suppress the immune system—such as cancer chemotherapy—warts can be a particular problem. You might hear all sorts of suggestions for getting rid of warts, from putting banana skins on them to burying a particular something in the garden. Some of these seem to work, and, although this is probably just the placebo effect, it still proves we don't really know how the immune system might be working!

Some evidence suggests that multivitamin and zinc supplement tablets will help to clear warts, and given these are fairly safe there is no harm in trying if you want to. Topical products can be used to shrink them down and reduce the keratin being produced, such as treatments available over the counter and online that contain salicylic acid. Freezing treatments—also called cryotherapy—can be effective, and involve a localized cold blast of something called liquid nitrogen onto the wart. There are some over-the-counter freeze treatments available, as well as a stronger type used in clinics. To work best cryotherapy needs to be repeated and aggressive, however, so the blistering it can cause is sometimes worse than the warts in the first place. Treatments for viral warts are not easy to access on the NHS, as most warts in healthy people will disappear over time without treatment.

There are also types of HPV linked to certain cancers, cervical cancer being the main example. Young people in the UK are now being offered an HPV vaccine; it targets the type of HPV linked to cervical cancer, and has led to a dramatic reduction in the number of new cases. There is a bit of evidence that it might also help people with skin warts too, so there may well be similar vaccines that protect against skin warts available in the future.

Bacteria

Bacteria are organisms with just one cell; they're larger than viruses and can survive on their own, although they generally like a host to live on too. There are millions of different types, but the ones that most commonly cause skin infections are called staphylococci and streptococci (sometimes just referred to as staph and strep) (Fig. 14.1).

Impetigo is a skin infection caused by staph or strep, which makes skin go red, crusty, and scabby. It can be treated with antibiotics, either in cream or tablet form, but you may well need a swab to check which bug is causing it before we can decide which antibiotic should be used. Overuse of antibiotics has meant that there are some difficult-to-treat bacteria left hanging around, so it's important to make sure you get the right treatment.

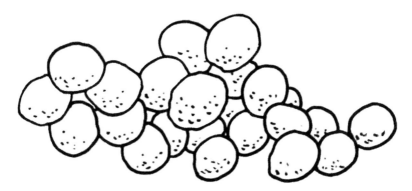

Figure 14.1 Staphylococci bacteria close up.
© Reproduced courtesy of Damian Hale.

Abscesses or boils are caused by infections deeper in the skin and are bigger than your average spot. They can be more likely to develop if you have an underlying health condition such as diabetes, but are often seen in young people with no apparent health problems. If you are getting recurrent abscesses then it's important to have a swab performed by your doctor, in order to check which type of bacteria is causing the infection.

Unlike impetigo however, abscesses are harder to treat with antibiotics; it can be difficult for them to get to the source of the infection, and so a lot of the time abscesses are opened up to allow the pus to drain out. Simple changes can also be helpful if abscesses keep reappearing, including washing with antiseptics and avoiding old, dirty razors that may be causing boils in areas you are shaving.

Cellulitis is a condition caused by bacterial infection in both the skin and the tissue underneath it. The skin turns hot and red, patients become quite unwell, and sometimes even need to come into hospital and have antibiotics via a drip.

Fungi and yeasts

Fungi and yeasts are a large group of organisms, ranging from tiny microscopic versions to big and (sometimes) edible mushrooms. It's the microscopic types that live on the skin, and a wide variety of them are found in our microbiome. For the most part they aren't an issue, but there are a few which can cause problems.

Fungi

Lots of different fungi are capable of causing skin, nail, or hair infections.

Fungal skin infections—sometimes called tinea—appear as red, scaly rings on the skin. This might explain why people also refer to the condition as 'ringworm', although confusingly it's not caused by a worm at all. The fungi that cause tinea are found on the top bit of the skin, where skin cells make the scaly stuff called keratin that these fungi live on. Antifungal creams and ointments are therefore usually enough to get rid of them, and it's important not to use corticosteroids; even though tinea can look a bit like eczema, the steroid creams used for eczema will make fungal rashes worse rather than better.

Tinea is more likely to appear in certain areas, and when it does it will sometimes be given a specific name. Tinea pedis is one of the best-known examples, often just called athlete's foot (Fig. 14.2). There is probably a certain amount of fungus on all of our toes, but the warm, sweaty places in between the toes are where these fungi grow best. When they get to be too much, tinea pedis develops, causing cracks in the skin, an itchy rash, and sometimes spreading to the nails too.

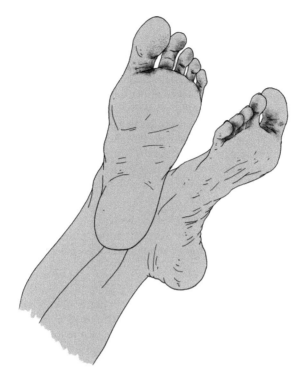

Figure 14.2 Fungal infection of feet—tinea pedis or better known as 'athlete's foot'.
© Reproduced courtesy of Damian Hale.

Fungal infections of the nails cause them to thicken and crumble. Some cases can disappear on their own, and others may respond to nail paints and creams; normally, however, if they are to be treated you need a tablet medicine. If the infection isn't causing you problems then a tablet might not even be recommended, because these medications aren't 100% effective and come with their own potential side effects. Terbinafine, for instance, is an antifungal tablet that can occasionally cause liver problems, and even though this happens rarely, it's still worth considering whether it's definitely necessary.

Tinea capitus is the name for fungal infection of the scalp, which can lead to inflammation and areas of hair loss. This might happen either in patches or larger areas, but it's important to pick up early because the hair loss can be permanent. Tinea capitus normally responds well to a tablet medicine taken for 4–6 weeks, and you may then consider using an antifungal shampoo to keep the infection away.

Yeasts

Pityriasis versicolor is a common rash caused by a yeast infection. It appears as pink spots, usually on the back, that can then fade to leave white or brown marks. These white marks can become more noticeable if you've been in the sun, and the infection itself seems to occur more during hot weather. Young people, those who exercise a lot, and possibly those who are particularly sweaty, are prone to developing pityriasis, but thankfully it is easy to treat. Just using a ketoconazole shampoo to wash the hair and body is usually enough, because the yeast lives on the scalp as well as the skin. It may still come and go at points, but the white marks should fade over time.

Malassezia is another yeast that lives on the scalp and face, and particularly likes the areas of skin with lots of grease-producing glands. A form of eczema called seborrheic dermatitis can be a problem in these places (Chapter 4).

Parasites

Parasites are living organisms that are able to move around, and pass from person to person by jumping between them. The small mites that cause scabies are a well-known example, as are lice. Evidence of lice have been found on Egyptian mummies, and it's likely that we've had lice around for the whole of human history.

Scabies

Scabies is caused by a very contagious parasite, which gives people an itchy, widespread rash. The mites responsible for it are pretty small, and can only really be seen with a magnifying glass. They live in little burrows between the fingers and around the genital area, and—even if you don't have a magnifying glass—you might be able to see the tiny red lines and bumps in these areas.

You only need a few mites on you to cause the rash, as the itchiness is the result of a kind of allergic reaction to the mite. If you're itchy all over then it's worth considering whether you might have scabies, and checking if anyone you are in close contact with is itchy too. The infection is transmitted easily, so all close contacts will need to be treated at the same time to stop the spread; it just involves a head-to-toe treatment, and you'll then need to clean your towels and bedsheets too. You may remain itchy for a week or two, but if you've used the treatment properly and not been reinfested this should settle down fairly soon.

Lice

Lice are big enough to see with just your eyes, so no need for a magnifying glass. All of them like hairy areas; some types prefer your head hair, whereas others are more often found in pubic hair. They can easily jump between people when we touch, for example, by putting our heads next to each other. There is some evidence that lice are now more common in older children for this reason, possibly because teenagers are more likely to crowd around phones, share tents at festivals, or wear their hair in certain styles.

It might feel a bit embarrassing to have lice, but it shouldn't. By definition, if you have them then you must have got them from someone; if you let people know then they can check and treat themselves too. Some of the stuff that claims to kill them doesn't work that well anymore, so the best way to deal with them is just to use a nit comb to catch the lice and their eggs. The eggs are called nits, and you'll need to keep combing wet hair for a couple of weeks to get rid of them. You can stop once you don't have any live lice or eggs left, and your scalp isn't itchy any longer.

Skin issues and bugs

Certain skin conditions—such as eczema and hidradenitis suppurativa—can make you more prone to infections (Chapters 4 and 7). On the other hand, however, other skin conditions, including psoriasis, might actually protect people from skin infections.

There are many other infections that can cause problems for the skin, not all of which have been covered here. If you have any other worries or questions then you should see your pharmacy or doctor to ask for advice. They can discuss the problem with you, and decide how best to manage things.

Resources

British association of dermatology information:
> https://www.skinhealthinfo.org.uk/condition/molluscum-contagiosum/
> https://www.skinhealthinfo.org.uk/condition/head-lice/
> https://www.skinhealthinfo.org.uk/condition/herpes-simplex/
> https://www.skinhealthinfo.org.uk/condition/scabies/

Part III

Living in your skin

15

Brain and skin

> **Key points**
>
> ◆ The time between 12 to 25 years old is key to brain development.
>
> ◆ Your attitudes to yourself and to society are changing during this period of development.
>
> ◆ People may feel really vulnerable around this time, and mental health issues can be a major problem. We also tend to learn loads during this period however, which can help us adapt to our world and develop resilience.
>
> ◆ Your skin and your brain interact in complicated ways, so it is important to manage both!

Your brain is a truly amazing thing. It's where all your thoughts and feeling start; it's in charge of every tiny movement you make, and controls the way you behave. Your brain is pretty much who you are.

It's a ridiculously complicated bit of kit, and we've spent centuries trying to unravel how it works. We know that certain parts of your brain have particular roles: some for movement, for example, some for memory, some for feelings. The development of new scanners and techniques to look at the brain has helped a lot in recent years, but there are still so many mysteries to solve.

The 'teenage brain'

We used to think that the brain stopped developing at the end of childhood, but it's now clear that this isn't true. While your brain doesn't grow much in size past this point, there are still loads of changes ongoing (Fig. 15.1).

Skin Conditions in Young People. Tess McPherson, Oxford University Press. © Oxford University Press 2021.
DOI: 10.1093/oso/9780192895424.003.0015

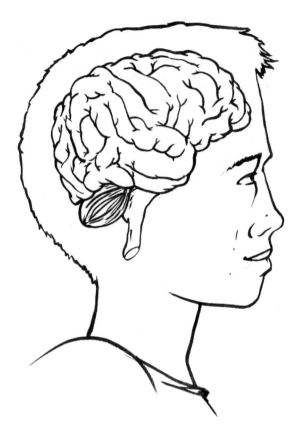

Figure 15.1 Your brain develops a lot during your teenage years.
© Reproduced courtesy of Damian Hale.

Lots of work has been done over the last few decades, with the help of scanners that can look at the amount of blood flowing to different parts of the brain. These have shown that certain areas, as well as the connections between them, are particularly busy during teenage years. This makes sense, as it's the time that you develop into an independent person, one that has to learn how to live in the adult world; no wonder there's so much going on in there. So, just as adolescence is a time for lots of physical changes, it's also a period of important mental development. It's no surprise, therefore, that these changes in your brain influence how you feel and act.

What is going on in your brain?

Your brain doesn't finish maturing until your mid-to-late twenties, although we're still not sure how it goes about doing this. The forming of active connections between brain cells seems to be particularly important in the process. One of the last areas to develop these connections is a section at the front of the brain, known as the prefrontal cortex; it's the area responsible for planning, prioritizing, and controlling impulses, which can really change over the course of adolescence.

Formation of these connections is likely influenced by loads of different things. Brain development is complicated, but there are particular themes that appear to have a critical impact at this age.

During adolescence, the following things tend to play an important role:

- **Socializing**—the way you behave with others, as well as the way you interact with the world in general, can have a big say in how you develop throughout adolescence.

- **Peers**—at this age, your peers will have huge influence over how you feel. Your brain can then be affected by these feelings—if you get the sense that you're not being included, for example—and this may impact on your mental health as a result. People your age will affect not just how you feel, but how you act too; adolescents behave differently around their peers, sometimes taking more risks than they would otherwise.

- **Risk**—adolescence is known to be a time when we take part in more risky activities, and this is why teenagers are more vulnerable to risk-associated injuries and deaths. Being aware of what is truly dangerous is vital, and acts to keep you safe. Taking some risks can be a good thing however; we all need to take risks at some point if we want to become more independent, and it can help your brain to learn.

- **Reward**—the parts of the brain that respond to exciting things are on high alert during adolescence, and this can encourage you to do things that make you feel good. It might mean your brain spends less time considering how this could impact on you and others, however, especially in the future.

- **Habits**—as your brain is changing so much, adolescence is one of the best times to learn. Habits started in your teens and twenties will likely continue into adulthood, so starting good habits—a good diet, exercise, healthy relationships—is great for the long term. On the other hand, habits such as smoking might be best avoided for the same reason; if you don't start, you won't continue.

♦ **Skills**—just as habits are easier to form, new skills are quicker to be picked up at this age. You've probably realized that you're generally a bit better at dealing with modern technology than older generations, for example. The adolescent brain is well prepared to adapt to our new, digital world, and can be affected by this technology in return.

The changes that happen in response to these influences can have knock-on effects, and making new connections between particular areas of the brain may not always be that easy. Dealing with these changes might mean anxiety and low moods are more likely, but it's important to remember that there are always upsides during what can be a really difficult period. Taking certain risks, for example, can help you to discover new and exciting things, and you have the opportunity to learn loads of things that will help you deal with the world that you're growing into.

The social brain

One really important development during adolescence seems to happen in the areas of the brain that are involved in something called 'social cognition'. This is just a fancy term for the way we understand and interact with others, and we do a lot of it without even really realizing.

When you see another person—at school, college, work, or just out-and-about—you will decide what mood you think they're in, and probably assume a bit about what they are like. You then use this information to guide how you interact with them. Your brain controls this process, without you really, consciously thinking about it. You constantly notice others, and because of this you tend to start wondering what they notice about you too. It seems adolescence is the time when all the processes involved in 'social cognition' start to really develop, and this can begin to make you feel worried about the way others view you.

Social exclusion

This 'social' part of the brain—along with all the hormonal changes you go through during puberty—can influence your mood. It's common for the way you look to affect this further. Fitting in and getting on with your peers seems really important at this time in your life, and you may feel like your appearance is key to this.

As we mentioned, the development of your 'social brain' can mean you're a bit vulnerable. It makes you a bit more conscious of the way other people see you, and you might find it harder to deal with feeling different or excluded too. This is where skin conditions sometimes become a problem, because they can make you even more aware of your appearance. If you're not happy with it, or you feel like it makes it hard for you to fit in, then it's really easy for your mood to be affected too.

Your skin and your brain

All your body parts connect and interact in some way, including the brain and the skin. Your skin and brain—along with all the other nerves that make up your nervous system—actually develop from the same starting blocks. There are cells involved in the early development of babies, while they're still in the womb, which can split off to become either brain cells or skin cells. It's pretty feasible that they could therefore be connected in some way, and there are actually some conditions present from birth than can affect both the skin and nervous system.

Throughout this book, we have stressed how closely tied your skin can be to your thoughts and feelings. We know having a skin problem that affects your appearance can easily alter your mood, but a skin condition won't just change your appearance; it could be itchy, it could stop you from sleeping, or it might mean you can't wear certain clothing. All this can have a big impact on the way you feel.

How does your brain play a role in things? Well, we know that certain feelings—stress, for example—can activate certain little chemical signals that circulate around your body, and these can then trigger inflammation. Lack of sleep has been shown to have a similar effect too. This is likely one of the reasons that skin conditions caused by inflammation, such as eczema, psoriasis, or acne, can flare up in people during times of stress.

Just as the brain can influence the skin in this way, it seems likely that inflammation in the skin could affect the brain in reverse too. Many of the common skin problems that we see in young people are chronic inflammatory conditions. As discussed in the various sections—and the glossary—inflammation is a response that involves the activation of many substances, and some of these substances can then become widespread throughout the body. More and more research is starting to show that inflammation in one area can actually have an influence on the whole body; while the visible problem might be on the skin, it's likely that more than just your skin is being affected. The changes to your thoughts and feelings could therefore be about more than just 'having a skin condition', as the inflammation caused by these conditions may actually be having a direct influence on your brain. This is an exciting theory, and studies should help answer the important questions it raises. Does

115

improving someone's mood clearly reduce the inflammation in their skin? Does treating the skin reduce inflammation in the brain, and thereby improve someone's mood?

Whatever the answer, it's really important to focus on managing not just your skin, but taking care of the way you feel too. Adolescence is a vulnerable time in terms of mental health, but it's also an opportunity. Show empathy, make connections, and look after each other; just make sure you're looking out for yourself as well (Fig. 15.2).

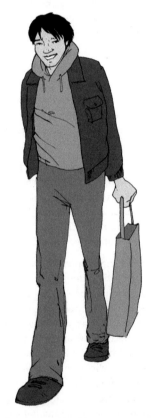

Figure 15.2 Taking care of your mental health is important, and could help your skin too.

© Reproduced courtesy of Damian Hale.

16

Skin and mental health

 Key points

* It's common for skin problems to affect your mental health, through a combination of how you feel it looks and how it feels.

* Psychodermatology is a word that refers to this interaction between your skin and your mental health.

* Sometimes mental health issues can cause problems for your skin too.

Mental health issues

These days, we hear so much more about the mental health of young people than we used to. The phrase 'mental health' refers to our thoughts, our feelings, and our behaviours, all of which are influenced by our brains. If everything is working as it should, then your thoughts and emotions—your 'mental health'—should be good too. If your thoughts or feelings are affected in some way, however, then—just as you can become physically unwell—your mental health might start to suffer.

As we mentioned in the last chapter, the brain is undergoing big changes during adolescence. All this change could explain why this is the time that many mental health conditions often emerge. Anxiety, depression, bipolar disorder, schizophrenia, and eating disorders are all examples that can develop in teenagers, and they seem to be more common than they used to be. This isn't necessarily because more people now have these conditions; it might just be that people are less frightened to be open about these things, which means more adolescents are getting proper diagnosis and treatment. The increase in discussion is a great thing, although while issues like anxiety and depression are talked about much more, others are still not being properly addressed. Conditions like schizophrenia, for example, aren't really spoken about as much, and can be very difficult for young people and their families to deal with.

Skin Conditions in Young People. Tess McPherson, Oxford University Press. © Oxford University Press 2021.
DOI: 10.1093/oso/9780192895424.003.0016

Mental health and skin

Another aspect of mental health that isn't often talked about is the effect that it can have on your skin. We've already discussed the complicated interactions between the brain and the skin, and also between the skin and the brain, in the previous chapter. These interactions are termed psychodermatology; the 'psycho' part refers to the brain, and the 'dermatology' part to the skin.

Psychodermatology involves a few different ideas, including that:

1. The skin conditions covered in this book can be exacerbated by stress—or other issues—in the environment a person lives in.

2. These skin conditions can lead to mental health problems, such as anxiety and depression.

3. Certain skin conditions may also develop due to problems involving the brain, or as a result of mental health issues.

The majority of this book discusses the first two of these ideas; the ways in which skin conditions can affect your thoughts, feelings, and actions. The next section looks at what can be done about this, and provides some general tips to keep on top of both your skin and mental health, whatever your skin condition.

The third idea—that skin conditions can actually result from mental health problems—is slightly different, but no less important. These skin conditions aren't due to a problem with the skin itself; instead, the skin problems are a result of behaviours that are influenced by your mental health. It doesn't necessarily have to be a known or diagnosed mental health problem to cause this kind of condition. What's important is to consider both the skin condition and any contributing mental health issues, diagnosed or undiagnosed, and this may require a dermatologist working alongside a mental health professional.

Ways in which mental health issues can cause problems with the skin

Compulsive hair pulling (trichotillomania)

Compulsive hair pulling is the recurrent, irresistible urge to rub or pull out hair, which therefore results in hair loss. Some young people find that pulling their hair makes them feel good, and that it relieves tension; they may also eat their hair after they pull it.

Compulsive hair pulling is more common in teenagers than younger children, with girls more often affected than boys. It's considered to be a type of obsessive-compulsive disorder (OCD), a mental health condition in which you have recurring thoughts or repetitive behaviours that you find difficult to control. These behaviours can range from habits such as nail-biting, to fixations on cleanliness and handwashing, for example. This kind of thing will have a massive impact, not just on your skin but on your entire life.

What can be done?

Hair pulling—and OCD in general—responds best to psychological support from a mental health professional. They guide people in using treatments such as cognitive behavioural therapy (CBT), which can be effective in helping them to experience their difficult thoughts or urges without performing the problematic behaviour. Medication can also play a role at times, particularly in severe cases.

People who develop patches of hair loss as a result of trichotillomania may also feel like they want to cover these areas; there is more information on this in Chapter 10.

Cutting (self-harm to the skin)

Self-harm happens when you hurt or harm your own body. It can be any kind of harm, although 'cutting' is one of the more common types; we see this most often in adolescent girls, and it usually involves cuts to the insides of the arms. The cuts tend to bleed briefly and then heal, with or without a scar, although if the cuts are deep they can cause serious problems.

Cutting may offer a temporary release of emotion, or make a person feel slightly more in control when they have difficult feelings that threaten to overwhelm them. If young people aren't able to find other ways to manage these difficulties however, then problems can develop; when those difficult feelings re-emerge, they may feel the urge to harm themselves again in order to feel better once more. Often, they will also hide the marks, due to shame or fear of attracting attention. This can mean that they rarely let health professionals know what's actually going on.

What can be done?

Please talk to somebody if you are struggling with cutting. It may be part of a mental health condition, it may not be; either way, there are loads of things that can be done to help. Many people need help in dealing with things over the course of their lives, and so learning how to manage your difficulties in a positive way can be a really useful life skill.

Scarring can be hard to deal with, especially if it's severe. Most young people want to cover these areas and this is absolutely fine. They should fade over time, but keeping your skin in good condition will help.

Medically unexplained skin lesions

Skin lesions caused by damage to the skin surface can present in a variety of ways, and will often look like other genuine skin conditions. Sometimes people will cause this damage themselves, although—unlike in self-harm—they won't be open about it or tell others that this is what has happened.

Dermatologists often call this condition dermatitis artefacta (DA). It's a term that implies that the skin conditions are artefactual—caused by people, rather than a specific disease—and is used to refer to skin problems where there is no underlying skin disease identified. It can really feel like you're being judged if anyone accuses you of damaging your skin, and we know that it's quite a complicated issue. It may not be intentional, and you might not even be aware that you are doing it. We prefer the term medically unexplained skin lesions or external skin lesions in order to avoid anybody feeling that they are being blamed.

If we take a sample of a skin lesion and look at it under a microscope, we can usually see what has caused it. Eczema, for example, would have a particular appearance associated with inflammation in the skin, as would psoriasis. In the conditions we're discussing here, however, if a sample of skin were taken it would not show any underlying skin disease. Instead, you would see changes that have been caused from the outside, for example, scratching or rubbing of the skin.

These kinds of lesions are found more commonly in girls; they may appear at any age, although are most frequent in early teenagers. They can often be confused with lots of other skin problems, in particular by health workers who do not see a lot of skin conditions. External skin lesions tend not to look or behave like inflammatory skin conditions, however, and so there are ways to tell them apart. The lesions often appear suddenly, and are usually in places that a person is able to reach on themselves. People sometimes rub or scratch their skin at night without realizing, for example, and so the lesions may then be present when they wake up.

We know that these types of skin lesions are often a response to emotional distress, or sometimes a result of psychological need. Unhappiness can present in the body in many ways; you may find that you get a headache when you're feeling stressed perhaps, or a stomach ache when you're sad. People can even have fits or seizures when they're feeling deeply unhappy or in need, despite not having any abnormality in their brain that would cause epilepsy. Our bodies are complicated things, with a nervous system spread throughout them. It's therefore not surprising that unhappiness and stress can lead to so many symptoms, and this may include skin lesions.

External skin lesions may be seen sometimes in young people who want others to think they have a skin condition. To some degree, they can find comfort in the attention that they get from other people including family and professionals; the attention might be focused on their skin rather than their thoughts and feelings, but it can feel good all the same. It may be a way of getting out of something they don't want to do, or it may be the only way they know how to ask for help. It could even be something they themselves are not really aware of; maybe it's happening when they rub their skin without realizing, or even just happening at a subconscious level. The problem can seem genuinely unexplained, which can be really frustrating.

What can be done?

It's important to explore any possible underlying explanation for the skin lesions that develop. Sometimes—but not always—tests will need to be done, to make sure there is genuinely no skin disease causing the lesions.

Focusing on supporting the way you're feeling is key, and this might be best done by a mental health professional. Alternatively, it could just be a trusted adult that you feel like you can confide in. Your skin can heal if no further damage is done to it, and the lesions will often settle down with the right kind of psychological support.

Recognize that your skin is sensitive. Any rubbing, scratching, or irritating substances can cause redness or grazes, so be careful to treat your skin as best you can. It can be helpful to use an emollient (Box 4.1) to soothe your skin.

It can also be helpful to consider whether you're aware of how these skin changes are developing, although not everyone will be.

Can you think of any triggers? Stress, for example? You may find that these develop at stressful times. It's also worth asking whether your skin lesions would prevent you from doing something you want to; or, alternatively, will they mean that you can avoid something you don't want to do? An awareness of these factors can allow you to start to address them, and to seek help for any anxiety, difficult thoughts, or worrying behaviours.

If you have found that having a skin condition means you can get out of doing something—school, for example—then try to be honest about this. Unnecessary medical appointments are not an easy way out, as they might lead to investigations that can be uncomfortable, as well as unnecessary treatments with unwanted side effects. Your health professionals can be most helpful if you are as open and honest with them as you can be. If you're struggling in any way, let them know; they should not judge you, and will be keen to help.

Coming up in the next section are some—hopefully—useful tips for looking after your mental health. Remember that if you're feeling low, you need to seek help. If things have got really bad and you're considering suicide, then this needs to happen urgently—speak to your GP, or consider calling 999 to get the help you need.

Resources

If you are struggling with your mental health then the websites below are great resources. All have urgent contact details:

> https://www.samaritans.org/
> https://www.mind.org.uk/
> https://www.rethink.org/
> https://www.childline.org.uk

17

How to be comfortable in your skin

 Key points

- Skin problems can impact on many aspects of your life.

- You are not the cause of your skin condition.

- You might feel like your skin condition is having a massive effect on you, but this can be dealt with; learning how to be resilient is an important life skill, and there are proven methods that help with this.

- There are various techniques that we can all use, in order to be more comfortable in whatever skin we have.

The impact of skin conditions

Having any kind of skin problem can affect you in multiple ways, and the extent to which it affects you doesn't always match up with how 'bad' the skin problem is. These things can sometimes seem small to other people, but may still have a massive impact on your life.

Thankfully, there are things we can do to improve almost any situation; not just treating the skin condition, but recognizing the wider impact that the condition is having too. This section describes some of the problems that skin conditions can cause for people, and looks at solutions that might be able to help.

How to be comfortable in your skin

When we talk about being 'comfortable in your skin', we're suggesting that you should be comfortable in both a physical and emotional sense. The previous sections have focused on improving the physical element of your skin

Skin Conditions in Young People. Tess McPherson, Oxford University Press. © Oxford University Press 2021.
DOI: 10.1093/oso/9780192895424.003.0017

condition, using treatments based on good evidence. Now, we'll look at how we can manage the impact skin conditions have on the way you feel.

Not unreasonably, a lot of young people feel that if their skin was OK—normal, unblemished, and not itchy or sore—then any associated problems they had would disappear. Treating the skin, especially these uncomfortable symptoms, is really important, and in fairness it will probably help with things like your mood and your stress levels. A lot of skin problems come and go, however, and even with treatment they won't be permanently 'cured'. This can leave people worried that their symptoms will flare up again, and these worries can be hard to shake off. As a result, most people will still have some skin-associated emotional issues, which are there even when their skin is clear or 'normal'.

So how can you deal with all this? It involves learning about how to help your skin, but also much more. You need to work out how to deal with uncertainty, to recognize the impact your skin has on your feelings, and to find the ways that help you cope. These are vital life skills; not just for living with a skin condition, but for dealing with all the inevitable ups and downs of life too.

Why me?

Lots of people ask, 'why me?', and that's totally understandable, especially if it seems like no one else has to cope with this kind of stuff. These feelings can also leave people feeling guilty for worrying about themselves when they know that there may be other people with worse skin or health problems. However, if something is affecting you do give yourself permission to ask these questions. It can sometimes feel really unfair that you have to deal with skin issues.

The answer to this: well, it's just as easy to ask 'why not someone else?' We're all different, and it's impossible to find an explanation for every single difference. We have strengths, we have weaknesses. We've got physical and mental attributes that we like, and almost all of us have some that we don't.

All of this applies to skin conditions too, because—as you've probably realized—most are complex disorders. It's hard to give a simple explanation for these differences in our skin, just as it can be difficult to say why some people are better than others at maths, at sport, or at art for example. The problem with skin, however, is that it's a lot harder to hide than these other insecurities. Lots of other people will be wondering why they find something hard, or wishing they could change something about themselves. You might not be able to see it, but every single person will have a 'why me? It's just worth reminding ourselves that we all struggle sometimes.

Uncertainty and control

Not knowing why you've got a skin condition can be really difficult, and people sometimes feel very angry or upset that it's not something they can control. Living with a skin problem that flares up unpredictably adds an extra level of uncertainty to your life too; your appearance can change without warning, and adapting to these changes can be really hard.

There is so much in life we can't control, and keeping these changes from happening is impossible. There are some things you are in control of, however, and it's these that we'll focus on now. The decisions you make about your lifestyle, what you do with your life, the way you see yourself, and the way you react to other people, are all things that you can choose to change if you want to.

Diet

Young people often ask about how food can affect their skin. It's a good question, but in general, eating the 'wrong' foods won't lead to any skin conditions. Unless you have a known allergy to a certain food, or a condition called coeliac disease—caused by a reaction to gluten—your skin problem won't be caused by the food you eat. There may be foods which you feel may flare you skin, for example, acne and eczema and this is covered in those chapters (Chapter 3 and 4).

Being a healthy weight is good for many reasons. Certain skin conditions— psoriasis and hidradenitis suppurativa in particular—can be worse the more you weigh. Your weight isn't the cause of the problem, as the conditions occur in people with healthy weights too, but losing weight might at least improve some of your symptoms and improve well-being in other ways. Eating food that contains fewer calories, as well as increasing the amount you exercise, is the best way to go about it; it's easier said than done a lot of the time, however, so ask for support if you need to. Remember not to overdo it, as becoming obsessed with your diet and losing lots of weight can actually be really dangerous. If you're not getting enough nutrients then this will be just as bad for your skin, and so it's all about trying to find the happy middle.

As long as you're making positive choices about your diet, you should be absolutely fine. In adolescence, you just need a good balanced diet in order to grow, and that should include all the major food groups: proteins, fats, sugars, vitamins, and minerals. It doesn't have to be too strict really, and for most people, a balanced diet simply involves eating what makes you feel good. This is an important thing to consider, as it does seem that what you eat can affect your mood. There are strong links between the gut and the brain, and so providing your gut with healthy nutrients can have a real positive impact on the way you feel. Fatty or sugary foods might make you feel good in the short term, especially if you're tired or stressed, but eating fruit and veg, nuts and seeds, and healthy proteins and fats, can give a long-term mood boost. You don't have to be obsessed, and it's fine to eat junk food sometimes; just try and keep your diet as varied and healthy as possible.

Eating is an important social activity, and it's something that you should enjoy. Get involved with cooking, eat with other people, and try not to stress too much about it. Small changes—rather than fad diets—could help your mood, and may improve your skin with it!

Exercise

Our bodies are made to move, and they feel better when they do. Research has shown that any extra movement we get during the day will have an impact on both our mood and health, and it doesn't have to be a huge amount; one study has shown that either 15 minutes of high intensity exercise, or 1 hour of low intensity exercise, can reduce the risk of depression. It could be literally anything: walking, running, cycling, swimming, or even just taking the stairs instead of the lift. As long as you enjoy it, it's a positive (Fig. 17.1).

Swimming is one activity that patients with skin problems commonly avoid. This is unsurprising, as swimming can involve exposing parts of your skin that you don't want to, and we know people may sometimes have had comments from others at pools about their skin condition. People making comments is not OK. The majority of conditions in this book—including eczema and psoriasis—aren't contagious, so there is absolutely no reason for you not to be there. Don't worry about getting your skin wet; sometimes it's not a good idea, but in the majority of cases it won't do any harm. Eczema, for instance, may even get better with swimming, as it's a good way to keep your skin clear of bugs that can aggravate your condition. So, get in the water. Or, if you don't fancy that, find another way to get active. Please don't let your skin stop you.

Outdoors and sunshine

There's loads of evidence that time spent in nature improves the way you feel, so why not move your exercise outdoors. Go join a park run, or even just take a walk in the park. You could maybe bring a dog along; either yours—or failing that—somebody else's. Listen to the birds, look at the trees, or climb a hill and soak up the view. It's a great way to get some perspective on the world.

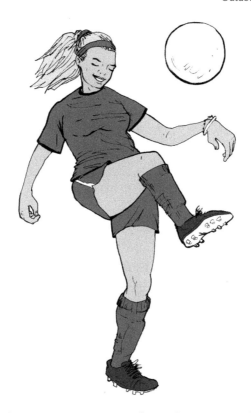

Figure 17.1 Doing exercise you enjoy is a good way to boost your mood and health.
© Reproduced courtesy of Damian Hale.

Sunshine is essential for your health; it allows your skin to make vitamin D, which is necessary for your body—and your bones in particular—to work properly. Sunlight can also help some skin conditions, and a form of light called UVB is sometimes used in dermatology clinics to treat psoriasis or eczema. However, too much is not good. Sunlight exposure over time causes your skin to wrinkle and age, and will increase the risk of you developing skin cancer when you get older. Skin cancer is very rare in young people, but getting burnt and using sunbeds—particularly if you're pale, or someone in your family has had skin cancer previously—causes problems further down the line. Wearing sunblock or a hat if you're out in the hot part of day can help keep your skin youthful. See Box 17.1 for more useful tips.

Box 17.1 Healthy skin for life: a few top tips

Whatever kind of skin you have, you want to do your best to keep it good working condition as you get older. Our skin ages over time and good habits, if started early, can help prevent this:

- Avoid sunburn and sunbeds

- Don't smoke

- Eat your fruit and veg

- Daily moisturizer—this keeps your skin barrier in good condition— there are plenty to choose between to suit your skin type

---

Smoking

Smoking is not good for your skin. It can increase the risk of certain skin conditions, and over time it will make your skin age and wrinkle. Vaping is probably a bit better, but it still isn't great. The fact that nicotine is incredibly addictive means it's really difficult to quit, so the easiest way to solve that problem is by never starting to smoke in the first place. If you are a smoker however, then it can feel impossible to get rid of the habit. It's one of the best things you could do for your skin though, so ask for help in quitting if you need it; there is absolutely loads on offer.

Alcohol and 'recreational' drugs

There are usually plenty of opportunities to experiment with substances that can influence your mood, and these are often tried during adolescence. Some of these are legal—although only from a certain age—whereas others are always illegal; their use can be associated with fines and prison sentences.

Most teenagers, although not all, will drink alcohol. Some will do it routinely before the legal age of 18, and a proportion of these will drink a lot. As with many things, a small amount of drinking is OK. Heavy drinking and binge drinking have been shown to have many negative consequences, however, from a short-term increase in accidents, to longer-term physical and mental health issues.

Alcohol can affect your skin as well as your mood, in that it can cause conditions such as psoriasis or eczema to flare in some people. Other recreational drugs can lead to specific problems for the skin too; cannabis, for example, can cause itchy skin, and an additive in cocaine called levamisole can trigger severe inflammation in the blood vessels that supply the skin.

Just remember that any substance that affects your brain may have both short- and long-term effects on you, some of which you don't always anticipate. These substances may also be illegal, which is a separate and important thing to consider. There are plenty of other places to get good advice on this if you're unsure about it all. Make sure you're making your decisions based on the way you want to live your life, not just doing things that your peers all claim to be doing.

Sleep

Although adults might call you lazy because you don't want to get up in the morning, or tell you that you're not a 'morning person', this probably isn't your fault. Science has shown that the levels of melatonin in the blood—known as the 'sleep hormone'—rise later at night in teenagers, which means they also come down later the next morning. This could explain why many young people stay up later and also why they might struggle with getting up the next day. Unfortunately, we all still live in a world that does require things to happen in daylight hours; you therefore have to learn to live through this period—when it can feel like you sometimes have jet-lag—and work on ways to get enough good quality sleep.

Young people actually need more sleep than adults, and should ideally get about 9–10 hours a night. Having sore or itchy skin can mean this is difficult however, making it more likely that you become sleep deprived. This could then affect you in loads of different ways; evidence suggests being short on sleep will lessen your immune system's ability to fight infections, as well as having a major impact on your mental health. You might then become more irritable and upset, act impulsively, find it harder to pay attention, and even be more likely to develop anxiety or depression.

If you're having a bad time with your skin which is affecting your sleep, then it's therefore really important to try and use treatments to improve things.

Whatever your skin is doing there are some simple, healthy tips that can help improve your rest (Box 17.2).

Tattoos and piercings

We do sometimes get asked whether it's OK to get tattoos or piercings. The answer is that there is a chance they could cause problems for the skin, so it's worth knowing about these before you consider one. Tattoos can be useful to take control of certain skin conditions—tattooing eyebrows in alopecia, for

---

Box 17.2 Tips for improving sleep

♦ Create some kind of wind down routine that works for you and try and make it regular.

♦ Get away from devices before and during sleep. The blue light acts like a 'wake-up call' (similar to having a shot of caffeine). Netflix have said their biggest competitor is sleep, so try not to let them win! It's also not the best time to be dealing with good or bad messages or news.

♦ Find time for some exercise or movement every day.

♦ Caffeine—the stimulant found in drinks such as coffee, tea, Red Bull, and Coke—is very good at keeping you awake. If you are finding it hard to fall asleep, don't have these 4–6 hours before bed.

♦ Try to make your bedroom dark, cool, and quiet.

---

example, or making a feature of a mark on skin. Although it's rare, tattoos can become infected or even cause allergic reactions, plus they're expensive and tricky to get removed if you decide you don't want them anymore. Piercings can also get infected or lead to scars, especially on the areas of skin prone to significant or bumpy scarring.

What you do to your skin is really up to you, but we would always recommend thinking seriously about it and make sure anything you have done is in a recognized place with good standards of hygiene.

How you see yourself

Making lifestyle changes similar to the ones suggested here can be really helpful, and will hopefully give you back a bit of control. Your attitude to all of this will be key in making you feel better, but perhaps even more important is the attitude you have towards yourself. When you've got a skin condition it can feel like other people are judging you sometimes, but—in my experience—the most negative influence often comes from you.

We all want more than to just fit in. We want to like how we look, and for others to see us as beautiful too. It's easy, therefore, to think that looking better will make us more likeable or loveable. People with skin conditions will often convince themselves that their skin makes them look ugly, however; they then try to hide their skin, stop wanting to see people, and become isolated and stressed. This is clearly really hard on a person's self-esteem.

So, how do we tackle all of this? It's about addressing the way you think about yourself, as well as the ways in which you think other people see you.

You

We know that we're all often our own biggest critics. Many people have negative thoughts about themselves, especially with regards to the way they look. You'd be surprised how supportive people can be if you're willing to talk about this kind of thing, because they may well be going through something similar too.

Sometimes it's worth asking whether you're being too hard on yourself. Take note of all your negative thoughts, and then try to quiet them. These voices might tell you that you're ugly, that your skin is bad, and that you don't deserve to be loved, but that's never true. There's no way you'd let anybody say that about any of your friends, so why should you say it to yourself? Defend yourself as if you're defending a friend, and you will realize that your negative voices are totally wrong.

Your parents and carers

Relationships between young people and their parents or carers can be complex, at any age really. Adolescence is the time when you transition from being a child—one who was probably fairly dependent on their parents or carers—to an independent adult, and this makes things even more complicated. It can be a pretty stressful period, and a skin condition may complicate things further.

As you to start to take more responsibility for what you do with your body and skin, there may be some strain on relationships. Parents can find it frustrating that they're not as involved in helping you care for your skin condition any longer. It's usually just because they care about you, but accepting that your life—and your skin—are becoming your own business might be something parents struggle with.

Some skin conditions tend to run in families. Parents may be understanding if they have—or used to have—a similar skin condition to you, but they will often also feel guilty if they think they've 'passed on' the skin problem. It's pretty unusual for young people to blame their parents for something that they may have inherited, however, and to be honest it's not really a useful thing to do anyway. There is very little we can do about our genes, so it's best to just try and concentrate on the good things we've inherited, and celebrate those instead.

We see many young people who are dealing better with their skin condition than their parents are. If parents are struggling, it's usually because they are worried. Often, they just want to know that you're OK. By showing and telling them that you're alright, you'll then be able to help educate and support each other. If you're not OK, however, then they will almost certainly want to help you; they might just be waiting for you to give them permission.

There's no one specific way that you should deal with your parents or carers concerns. Just try and see things from their point of view, and encourage them to see things your way too. It will probably be good for your relationship, and may help you at the same time.

Education and work

How your skin is can affect attending school, college, university, and work. Depending on the problem there should be appropriate support for this. Speak to your doctor or school or college nurse to make sure they know what you are dealing with. They should be able to make sure that you have appropriate support and there may be specific concessions for applications or exams.

Essentially a skin problem shouldn't stop you doing anything you want to do with your life. However, it may make you think more carefully about choices. The military does exclude applications for people with health conditions including skin problems. If you have very sensitive skin or eczema, then a job which involves lots of contacts with irritating substances like hairdressing or health-work may make it more difficult to manage your skin. However, there should always be roles you can comfortably do so please don't rule anything out without talking to someone first.

Other people

The world brings you across thousands of people during your day-to-day life. Many people can be kind, non-judgemental, and accept you whatever is going on with your skin. Some people may try to reassure you that 'it doesn't look that bad' which doesn't always feel very helpful if you don't believe that is true. Most sadly some people can react to skin disease in really unhelpful ways. I've had patients who've been asked to leave swimming pools, for example, because of ideas or views wrongly held by others. These other people may experience a built-in fear of skin problems without even realizing, because in centuries gone by, skin disease was more commonly infective. Conditions such as syphilis and scabies are a lot less common these days, however, and most chronic skin problems are now not infective and therefore cannot be 'caught'. Negative attitudes from the past remain though, and this can create problems.

We know that having a skin problem can affect your close relationships and make people feel concerned about developing intimate relationships in some cases. However, we see for the most part that true friendships and strong relationships will not be affected by having or worrying about a skin conditions and hopefully this book will help with this.

Part of our work as dermatologists involves educating the world, and trying to encourage more accepting and supportive attitudes towards skin problems. Patients with skin conditions might not realize, but they can be really helpful in achieving this goal. We see patients who are happy to expose their skin, both online and offline; it seems scary, but it makes it easier for others to understand certain skin conditions, and to learn to be kinder as a result.

Social media

There's a lot said about the influence of social media on mental health. The thing about seeing everybody's lives online, is that it encourages us all to compare ourselves. Often, we only see people's 'best life'—and 'best skin'—however, because they've carefully chosen what they put on social media. Social media can be used to project a 'self-image' by lots of us. Posting pictures may feel like the last thing you want to do if you don't think your skin looks good however, and it can really get people down. Comparing yourself to this probably won't make you feel great at first, so it's important to start to try and understand your relationship with social media (Fig. 17.2).

There's evidence that lots of people spend time on sites that make them feel less good about themselves, even though they're well aware of how this affects them. The first thing to do is to recognize that there are downsides to social media. All the comparisons to other people might damage your self-esteem, and in some cases make you feel that you should try and change your appearance in ways that are not possible or sensible. The demand for unnecessary cosmetic surgery has grown massively in young people recently, which is definitely a cause for concern. Nasty comments from other people can make things even worse, and you might find that people are sometimes a lot meaner when they're hidden behind a computer screen.

The other catch with spending loads of time online is that you'll have less time to other things, especially exercise and sleep. It's worth knowing that social media companies use people as products, and they design apps that keep you clicking and scrolling in order to fuel their business.

Having said all this, a healthy relationship with social media can be achieved. There's growing evidence that if it's used as a tool to make genuine connections, it can be a positive influence. It allows us to hear from positive people

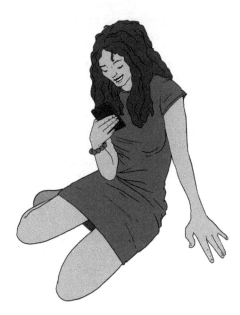

Figure 17.2 Developing a healthy relationship with social media can help your confidence, focusing on connections not comparisons.
© Reproduced courtesy of Damian Hale.

with powerful messages, and to provide support for one another. You can take control of this, using what you want in the way that is best for you. Maybe consider turning off notifications at times, or keeping away from your phone when you're doing something else; that way you're only on social media when you actually want to be.

Dealing with judging, staring, and bullying

Looking 'different' can mean that people view you differently as a result. It's ridiculous, it shouldn't happen, but you can be judged for your skin. If this ever happens, then please just remember that the people who judge you negatively are generally not worth bothering with anyway.

Staring

Looking is OK; staring is not. In fairness, there's always a chance that someone might be looking at you for another reason. They may be talking to you, or even just looking in your direction. If you feel like they've been looking at your skin a bit longer than normal however, the first thing is to remember that humans are naturally curious creatures! We all tend to glance for slightly longer at something or someone that we don't often see.

People may not know what your skin condition is, and therefore be concerned for you. Some people, especially younger children, may stare without even realizing they are doing it. Try and tell yourself that it's OK for people to look, especially if they are being friendly. If you think someone is staring at you then you could try giving them a quick smile. It lets them know that you've seen them staring, and will make most people feel embarrassed enough that they stop staring straight away.

You don't need to talk about your skin if you don't want to, and you shouldn't feel obliged to explain it to anyone. If people do ask—or stare—it may help to have a stock answer that assures people you're okay (Box 17.3). Then you can get on with talking about other things.

Bullying

Bullies are people who try to harm or intimidate others that they think are vulnerable. It can happen in person or more commonly online. Online or 'cyberbullying' may start because, when people can stay anonymous on the internet, they feel like they can get away with saying things they wouldn't ever say in person. This can be dangerous. We know that these kinds of comments can really affect young people with skin problems; they may have gone online just to look for some support, and instead have to deal with people saying hurtful things about their skin condition. It's easy to view bullies as people with power and control, but we all know that it's complicated; someone who wants to pick on other people's weaknesses often has a real place of weakness within themselves. Why else would they feel it was necessary to intimidate people otherwise?

Knowing this still doesn't make it all that nice to be bullied, in person or online, but it can help to understand that it's not your fault. What's wrong with being perceived as being vulnerable anyway? Showing our vulnerabilities is a form of strength, and it takes a brave person to do so.

Nobody deserves to be bullied. If you are being bullied then it is best not to fight or bully back, and definitely not helpful to keep it to yourself. Always tell someone you feel comfortable talking to and get help in sorting it out properly.

Box 17.3 Explaining your skin condition

Here are some tips that might help explain skin problems and alopecia to others:

Acne

'Everyone gets spots—mine are quite active at the moment. You probably already know this, but we don't get them just because we're dirty or unhealthy.'

Eczema

'My skin gets red and itchy because of my eczema; it's not infectious though.'

Psoriasis

'My skin gets patches of inflamed skin on it sometimes. It's called psoriasis, and it's not infectious; it's fairly common actually.'

Vitiligo

'My skin is pale due to a condition called vitiligo. It doesn't make me ill, and other people can't catch it.'

Alopecia areata

'I have an autoimmune condition that affects my hair, which is why I've got patches missing. It doesn't make me ill, and it's not infectious.'

Or, if you don't want to talk about it . . .

'I don't really want to talk about my skin/hair today.'

Alternatively, just change the subject to anything else you want to talk about; something you're interested in that has nothing to do with your skin, your hair, or your appearance.

How your skin condition makes you feel

Having a skin problem feels rubbish sometimes. It can affect your self-esteem, your relationships with others, and—if it comes with the staring and bullying that we mentioned—it can be really difficult. It's important to recognize that these kinds of things can be pretty stressful, and you may feel down sometimes. Thankfully there are things you can do to help make this a bit easier, and there are always people you can turn to for support.

Stress

In the previous chapter, we talked about the ways in which stress can affect your skin. You shouldn't feel like your stress has caused your skin problem, because there are loads of really stressed people around who have no skin problems at all. You aren't responsible for the development of your skin condition. Stress doesn't help your skin however; it can get you down, it can make you anxious, it can stop you sleeping, and all these things may make you feel like your skin is getting worse. This can start a vicious cycle, where you become even more stressed out by your skin and it starts all over again.

Sometimes, stress is a positive thing. We all need a bit of stress to get us to work for an exam, or to perform in sport, and in these cases channelling the stress can be a useful tool. Stress can clearly be negative too though—especially when it comes to skin—and learning ways to handle your stress is therefore an important life skill. Relaxation techniques and breathing practice (Box 17.4) can help in the short term, as can finding activities that make it easier for you to switch off. Recognizing and talking about your feelings is also really useful, and is something that you can carry on doing long term.

Your mood

We know that young people with skin problems have higher levels of anxiety and depression, as well as more suicidal thoughts. Everyone's mood goes up and down, and this is to be expected; usually it's just a reaction to what's going on in your life at the time. If you feel low most of the time, however, or if you can't feel positive about things and enjoy them like you used to, then these could be the signs of a mental health condition such as depression. There's a lot of evidence that mental illness is—and always has been—a big problem in teenage years, so it's very important to take how you are feeling seriously. The first thing to do is to recognize that you are struggling, then talk to someone in order to get support quickly.

Get help

If you are struggling with low mood, or feel like you can't cope; if you've decided life isn't really worth living, and are reading this thinking that it is all pointless—you likely need someone to help. Depression is an illness, and it requires treatment just like any other condition. Sometimes you can support yourself, and keep on top of your mood and stress levels using the strategies and resources in this section. At other times, however, you might need help from a professional. We understand that it can feel like a big deal for some

---

Box 17.4 Breathing techniques

We all need to breathe, and the way we breathe can actually be really important. Focusing on your breathing when you're feeling bad can be a great way to help calm yourself.

Example 1

If you're feeling anxious or panicky, then slow your breathing down for a few minutes.

Fill your lungs.

Wherever you are and whatever you are doing, try to centre yourself. Ideally stand, or if you're sitting then just place your feet on the ground. Breathe, and feel your breath move all the way down your body and into your feet. Do this for 10 breaths, and feel yourself start to calm down.

Example 2

1. Inhale deeply through your nose, and expand your stomach outwards while counting to 4. Feel the breath reach its way throughout your body.

2. Hold your lungs full of air for another count of 4.

3. Exhale through your nose—not your mouth—while contracting your tummy inwards for 4 seconds. Feel all your stress released with that air.

4. Hold your lungs empty while counting to 4.

5. Repeat for 1–5 minutes.

Deep breathing techniques like these can be used when you're not feeling great, and if you keep practising then it can help to keep you in a calmer place. It's been shown that focusing on your breathing for just 2 minutes a day can reduce your levels of anxiety, which should also improve the way you feel.

---

people to admit that they need help, and often it seems difficult to work out where to get it from. Remember that help is much easier to give if you ask for it, and there are services that are there whenever you need.

We have good evidence that psychological therapies or medications can be useful in these situations. Some of the different types of 'talking therapies' are listed next, and may help you in dealing with low mood and anxiety if it becomes a problem. The idea is that they encourage you to try and do the things you are avoiding because of what your thoughts are telling you. For example, if you are feeling like no one likes you, then you are more likely to be isolated in your room, which can contribute to you losing touch with your friends and make you feel even less liked by others. In a similar way, the treatments will aim to help you get back to all the activities you used to do again.

Sometimes medications can also help, although they are often most effective when used alongside talking therapy. A family of medicines known as selective serotonin reuptake inhibitors (SSRIs) are most commonly used, but your doctor will help you to assess which is best for you.

Psychological techniques to help with skin problems

There are several proven ways to improve your mood or change your behaviour, using psychological techniques that many patients find helpful. They involve training your brain to develop more healthy pathways, which can then prevent you from feeling low or worrying unnecessarily. Some people think they're great, others find that these kind of thinking techniques aren't helpful at all; it's absolutely fine either way. We've briefly described some simple versions of these techniques here (Box 17.4), and you should be able to access them in more detail through teams that offer psychological support.

Mindfulness

Mindfulness has become very popular in recent years, and has been found to work well for some people with long-term conditions such as eczema and psoriasis. It basically involves focusing your attention totally on what's going on in your present. When we are being mindful, we are fully engaged in whatever we are doing at that moment and, although we are aware of all our thoughts and feelings, we are not getting caught up in them.

It might be done at the same time as breathing techniques (Box 17.4), or with various types of meditation. Many people have a structured 'meditation practice', but there are other ways of practising mindfulness; if you fancy having a go, there are several good online resources that can help.

Habit reversal

Habit reversal training is a treatment that we use to address repetitive behaviours, such as you scratching your itchy skin (Box 4.3). It involves you building an awareness of the urge you have to carry out the habit, and then learning how to put up with it without giving in! You might do this by focusing on something else, employing relaxation techniques, or doing something that makes the behaviour difficult; playing with a stress ball or a game on your phone instead of scratching your skin is a good example.

Cognitive behaviour therapy (CBT)

CBT looks at how your thoughts and feelings affect your behaviour, and has been found to be a very effective way to treat a wide range of mental health issues. It encourages you to become aware of the unhelpful ways we sometimes think about situations, and to see how these thoughts can affect your mood and the way you behave. By identifying and challenging these unhelpful thinking patterns and behaviours, you can change the way you feel and what you do.

As well as being an effective treatment for low mood and anxiety, CBT can also help with the self-consciousness and loss of confidence that often arises when someone has a skin problem.

Acceptance and commitment therapy (ACT)

ACT is a mindfulness-based therapy. It aims to change the relationship we have with our difficult thoughts and feelings, allowing us to be open to them rather that fighting or avoiding them; this can then help us to live a more full and meaningful life. ACT has been found to be effective for a wide range of psychological and physical health problems.

Don't be defined by your skin

We've talked a lot in this chapter about the lifestyle changes that might help your skin, and the techniques that you can use to look after your mental health too. The suggestions we've made are based on scientific evidence, and so there's a good chance that at least some of them will work for you.

Great life advice doesn't always have to be based on science though; people learn so much through experience, and you probably know more about how it feels to live with your skin condition than a scientist or researcher ever could. These last few pages just contain a few tips and tricks that have helped people deal with their skin problems before, and will hopefully remind you that you're not on your own. Lots of people have skin conditions, but nobody should be defined by them—there's so much more to you than your skin.

Acceptance

One of the best—but often hardest—things that you can do for yourself, is to just accept who you are. This doesn't mean resigning yourself to having to deal with things that are unacceptable, or struggling alone with your problems. Instead, it involves learning about yourself and being able to live with that; accepting the things that you can't—and maybe don't need—to change.

The saying that 'beauty isn't skin deep' is true. There's so much more to you that you can learn to love, and as you start to see that, you might even begin to love your skin too. The marks and scars on your skin are unavoidable, but they still tell a story. In Japan, they celebrate this idea with a tradition called kintsugi; it involves using golden glue to repair the cracks in broken china, embracing the flaws and the imperfections. As you go through life, it's picking up these kinds of scars that makes you beautiful.

Exposure

It's not your responsibility to feel more confident, or to 'be more amazing'. Everyone else should respect you for who you are, and accept the skin you're in.

As you start to accept your own skin however, you could try showing it to the world. People are actually less likely to react than you might think, because they're usually wrapped up in their own worries and issues. Challenge yourself to go swimming, or just get outside and see what happens; often no one even notices. Plus, if they do—so what?

Avoid avoidance

You shouldn't let your skin rule your life. We see many patients who shy away from activities, or avoid doing things that they would likely enjoy; some even avoid important, potentially life-changing things, like job interviews, parties, and meeting new people.

Don't wait for your skin to clear up before arranging to do things, and try not to avoid doing things if your skin is feeling or looking bad. There may be times when you want to hide, and everyone wants to hide sometimes. It can feel like a big challenge, but just remember to keep going, because not missing out on those vital life opportunities is so important.

One of the main things that motivates me to work, and to support young people with skin problems, is that I've seen some of my older patients with chronic skin problems unable to live their lives to the full. They would have had richer lives if they had felt less need to hide. It usually started early, with them avoiding small things, before their lives then became stuck and they got trapped in an avoidance cycle. All this time they have missed opportunities, and no longer feel able to change things. That's why you need to get out of the avoidance cycle now, while you still have your whole life ahead of you.

Connection

Getting out and seizing these opportunities is a huge part of being human. We're a tribal species, and so we thrive off the connections we make through doing this. It relies on shared experiences, shared feelings and ideas. It's the sense of belonging to something bigger than ourselves.

When you do anything with other people, eat together, volunteer to help them, or even just watch something; when you open up and talk about your feelings, or find you have something in common—then you're experiencing connection.

The world we live in has been designed to create more connections than ever before, yet somehow, the 'digital age' can often make these connections feel less genuine. In order to properly connect with people, we have to give our time and our honesty. We don't connect with each other by trying to earn approval and compliments, or by establishing superiority. It can often feel like social media is full of this kind of stuff, but when it's used as a genuine way to stay in touch it can actually improve your mental well-being. Support groups, which allow you to share experiences of your skin with others, have been shown to help with this. These connections can be made in loads of ways, and some of the strongest are formed through supporting others.

Support

Support can be found in lots of places. Some find that being with others who have similar problems can be helpful, although these types of support groups are not for everyone. You may not want to share your story with others, or to hear about their problems too. Increasing numbers of online sites and forums are available however, which mean you don't have to physically attend a meeting where you might feel uncomfortable or exposed.

Many online resources—healthtalk.org, for example—provide recordings of other young people talking about their skin conditions. They've been shown to make people feel less alone in dealing with their problems, by demonstrating how others have struggled and found solutions.

You could even think about supporting others; it doesn't necessarily have to be skin-related either. Are there support groups you can play a role in? Are there elderly people who need help? Assisting others, in any way, has been shown to improve both mental and physical health, and research has revealed that committing an act of kindness—once a week, over a 6-week period—is associated with an increase in well-being. Connecting with others, especially those who need help, can be both great for them and rewarding for you. It might make you feel a bit better about yourself, and could put what you are dealing with into perspective.

Being grateful

People often talk about having a 'positive mental attitude' (PMA), but what actually is that? And does it really help?

I don't buy into a narrative that says, 'if you are positive, bad things don't happen'. This can be a slippery slope. People might blame themselves for getting a disease, or for their disease getting worse, just because they weren't being 'positive' enough. That's unhelpful, because we know that there is no good evidence to say that this is the case. Skin conditions are complex processes and so if you're struggling, you shouldn't feel responsible.

Unfortunately, bad things do happen to good people. It is OK to feel like things are a bit unfair because yes, it can feel unlucky to have a skin problem; in a way, it is. Self-pity can be dangerous however, and getting hung up on this probably won't be that helpful. People who identify as unlucky tend to approach life in an 'unlucky' way, and it's been shown that they don't notice opportunities because they're too busy focusing on the bad stuff. Starting to concentrate on the positives will mean that life can begin to open up; you'll see more opportunities, take more opportunities, and more good things will happen as a result. It may feel difficult, but we know that people can, and do, change their approach to life in positive ways. This may not always clearly improve their skin, but it definitely improves their life experience.

One way to help build a PMA is simply to think of something you are grateful for each day. You could do it first thing in the morning, last thing at night; whenever works best for you. It doesn't have to have anything to do with your skin, although some young people do grow to realize that their skin problem can sometimes have a positive influence on their lives. It could just be your friends, your family, or the weather; perhaps just doing OK in a test, or the fact that someone said something nice to you that day. Even if you think it's been rubbish, there will always be at least one small thing each day that you can be grateful for.

Meaning and value

Work out what gives your life meaning and—as long as it's legal and safe—keep doing it! (Fig. 17.3).

You don't have to be the best at it, or even any good at it all, just as long as it means something to you. The list is endless: socializing with friends, sport,

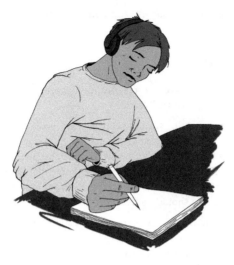

Figure 17.3 Find something you like doing and keep doing it.
© Reproduced courtesy of Damian Hale.

work, drama, music, dancing, cooking, eating, writing, drawing, reading, gaming, your pet. Everyone has something that means something to them, or an activity that suits them and that they enjoy doing. It will be different for all of us, and you may have to try a few things out before you find yours. Any activity that focuses your attention and lets you clear your mind a bit is good; it should hopefully let you lose yourself in what you're doing.

The bigger picture

Sometimes it's worth just getting things into perspective. Spend a moment, wherever you are, and imagine looking down on yourself from the ceiling. Then go further, and imagine seeing yourself from the sky: among all the other millions of people, with all their different skins. Moving around, getting on with their stuff, worrying about their lives, and possibly even coping with skin problems like yours.

Now go further still, and imagine you're looking down on the earth from space. We share this world with over 8 billion other people and over 2 billion different species of life, and from this distance, each of us is just a tiny speck on it. That might make you feel a bit insignificant, but maybe it helps to put our individual problems into perspective too. Just the fact that we get to be alive and a part of this universe is crazy enough in itself, and it's hopefully something worth being grateful for.

Going forward

It's a changing world that we live in, and taking responsibility and developing resilience is important in helping you cope. Growing up with any kind of problem can make you better at getting through life, and skin conditions are no exception. This is what young people have to say about it:

'I'm almost proud of my psoriasis, to be like: "What's wrong with it? Like if you've got a problem with it, I don't really want to hang out with you."' (Female age 16)

'Obviously, like if I hadn't had it (eczema) in the first place I'd be . . . I actually think I'd be such a different person today, if I hadn't been as confident as I am now; like pick myself up from it, and fight against. I think my confidence is probably actually up on the fact that I've suffered eczema, in a weird way.' (Male age 18)

'I think in a weird way, it's actually made me more confident. Because, since it's got better, I've now been like, 'two fingers to you, eczema' and am taking back my life.' (Female age 17)

Final thoughts

Accept your skin and who you are.

Live each moment, and each day, to the full.

Love each other.

Love yourself.

And try to be a bit kinder, to yourself and to others.

Take care of yourself.

Be comfortable in your skin.

And when you're truly comfortable in your skin?

Not everyone will like you.

And you won't like everyone either.

But you'll be able to get on with your amazing life.

Appendix

Additional resources

Accessing care

If you live in the UK, you are entitled to care provided by the National Health Service (NHS). For all those eligible for NHS services, treatment is free at the point of delivery; this means there is no need to pay for any appointments, with GPs or with specialists, or for any procedures and treatments approved and funded in the area where you live. Most people pay a small fixed fee for their prescription medications, although if you are under 18—or in full time education—you are exempt from this. Further procedures, including light treatment and surgery, are then fully covered for everyone. It should be noted however, that procedures considered to be 'cosmetic'—such as the removal of harmless skin lesions or moles—may not be offered by the NHS.

If you want to ask for advice about a skin complaint, the first step would be to make an appointment to see your registered GP. You can make an appointment at a time and date that suits you and, as long as they have an available slot at the time, you can specify the GP you want to see. Depending on your GP practice, you might have a choice of ways to get in touch; by email, through the practice website, or by phoning or calling in. They may then offer different ways to have that appointment, either face-to-face at the GP practice, by speaking on the phone, or via a video link.

If your initial appointment isn't a face-to-face one, you may be asked to send in a photograph of your skin complaint. You should not be asked to do this if the skin problem is in a sensitive area, around the breasts or genitals for example, and you do not have to do it if it would make you would feel uncomfortable in any way. Whatever you decide, make sure to talk to your GP first before agreeing to send any photos. It's also worth remembering that you can take someone to part—or all—of your appointment if you want to, whether it's face-to-face or over the phone.

The GP might suggest a treatment plan, and then ask you to come back in a few days or weeks. It is important to make a follow up appointment after trying a medicine, because if any change to your treatment is needed this can then be arranged. The GP might also want you to see a skin specialist (dermatologist); when they first meet you perhaps, or after there has been time to see whether the initial treatments they suggested have worked. If that is the case, then they will arrange a referral for you. You might have a choice of places to have your appointment, but be prepared for the possibility that you have to wait for this to come through. Your GP will be able to help if there are any difficulties, and—unless it is one of the medicines that can only be given to you by a dermatologist—can continue to provide prescriptions for your treatments after you have been seen by specialist care.

Resources and bibliography

Online resources are listed in chapters for specific conditions

Some general skin resources

https://www.skinhealthinfo.org.uk/—British Association of Dermatologists—Patient information leaflets and useful links for many skin conditions

https://www.britishskinfoundation.org.uk/—UK charity focused on skin health and research into skin conditions

http://healthtalk.org/peoples-experiences/skin-conditions—healthtalk.org is a patient experience website covering many different conditions and a valuable resource for different experiences. Section on skin conditions affecting young people (eczema, psoriasis, acne, alopecia)

http://bspd.org/adolescent-dermatology/—British Society of paediatric dermatology section on adolescent skin with more resources on both common and rare skin conditions

https://www.ypfaceit.co.uk/—Online support for young people with conditions or injuries affecting their appearance

https://www.dermnetnz.org—New Zealand based website with clear and well-informed articles on many skin conditions. Aimed primarily at healthcare workers, so uses medical language

https://www.hse.gov.uk/skin/employ/index.htm—Information on skin and employment

Glossary

Acitretin *See* Retinoids

Acute A process which is short lived.

Adrenaline autoinjector Commonly called Epipen. Used in severe allergic reactions as adrenaline can be effective to calm down allergic response.

Alitretinoin *See* Retinoids

Androgens Steroid hormone with many effects; responsible for male characteristics in humans. Biological females have androgens although at lower levels. They are mostly made in testes, ovaries, and adrenal glands. Anabolic steroids is a group which includes natural androgens like testosterone and also man made (synthetic) androgens used by cheating athletes and some body builders.

Antiandrogen Medication which blocks or partially blocks effect of androgens

Antibiotics Medicines designed to target bacteria. Some antibiotics are used largely for anti-inflammatory effects on the skin rather than treating infections and may be taken for longer than a normal 'course'. Care needs to be taken not to misuse antibiotics as there is growing problems with bacterial resistance in the world.

Antihistamine Medications that block histamine.

Anti-inflammatory Any treatment which targets inflammation.

Antiseptic Substances that reduce bacteria. Different from antibiotics as work to weaken and slow growth of bacteria and other infectious agents rather than kill (antibiotics, antifungals, antiparasitic, etc.). As bugs do not seem to develop resistance to antiseptics they are safer to continue long term.

Apocrine glands A type of 'sweat gland' in skin of armpit, eyes, and nipples which open into the hair follicle and release scented substances, causing the smell of sweat.

Atopic Inherited tendency to over-react to normal things in the environment. Being atopic means an increased risk of atopic eczema, atopic rhinitis (hay fever), asthma, and food allergies. Some people will have all and some will have only one or two from the atopic package!

Autoimmune The process of the immune system targeting 'self' rather than external agents (which is what it is really supposed to do). The reasons for autoimmune conditions are complex and tend to run in families.

Blister Pocket of fluid in the skin. Many causes of blisters including friction, burns, and also inflammation in the skin.

Chronic Any process which lasts a long time. This does not mean severe and most chronic conditions will fluctuate in severity. Many chronic conditions do not have a 'cure'—this means they will not disappear for ever but may well be totally controllable.

Corticosteroids A type of steroid which can have wide-ranging anti-inflammatory effects.

Eccrine glands A type of 'sweat gland' which opens directly onto the surface of skin and present all over body including areas without hair like palms and soles (where they may be particularly active).

Emollient A fancy name for moisturizer, which can be helpful to treat any dryness in the skin.

Evidence-based Using evidence from clinical trials to make decision on the most effective and safest treatments to use.

Hair follicle The skin pore with a hair growing out of it. We have trillions of these of these on our skin!

Histamine Chemicals released by cells which are part of an immune response. These can be released by mast cells in the skin due to an allergy or insect bite but may be released without an allergic trigger. Histamine release causes itching and swelling.

Inflammation Inflammation is caused by increased activity of the immune cells in your body.

Isotretinoin *See* Retinoids

Keloid A scar which is lumpy and can be itchy. Any scar can keloid but risk areas are the upper chest and back. Keloids are more common in black skin and can run in families.

Keratin/Keratinocytes/Keratinization The skin cells in the top layer of skin are called keratinocytes. These cells make keratin. Keratin is a tough substance responsible for structure of skin and also hair, hooves, and horns. If keratinocytes are too active this can cause the skin to get 'scaly' = the dry stuff on the skin.

Long acting Effects last for longer. Typically, longer than 4 hours and for some medications, can be weeks or longer.

Non-sedating Does not make you feel sleepy.

Oral contraceptive pill Pill that works on female hormones prevent ovulation and therefore risk of pregnancy. There are various types.

Pigment Different shades of colour of skin. Pigmentation of skin depends on the number and activity of melanocytes in the skin and there are thousands of variations in this. Our skin pigment can affect how easily we burn in the sun and what difference skin conditions look and how the skin looks following inflammation. Hypopigmentation is reduced pigment in the skin and hyperpigmentation is increased pigment in the skin—processes often caused following inflammation in the skin. Depigmentation is complete loss of pigment as can be seen in the condition Vitiligo.

Placebo effect Benefits of medical intervention not explained by property of treatment itself. Placebo effect can be pretty high, sometimes almost as high as some effective medications—showing the importance on expectations and beliefs in how treatments work.

Port wine stain Birth mark caused by changes in the blood vessels. Can be anywhere on body but particularly common on the face.

Retinoids A class of medications related to vitamin A. This is the same vitamin found in carrots but in retinoid medicines is much more concentrated. They have actions on various processes in the skin including the pilosebaceous unit (Isotretinoin in acne) and the scaliness of the skin; a process called keratinization (Acitretin and Alitretinoin).

Scale Causes by the cells in the top layer of the skin called keratinocytes making keratin. Seen in fungal infections, eczema, and psoriasis.

Sebaceous glands Tiny glands attached the hair follicle = pilosebaceous units.

Sedating Can cause drowsiness.

Short acting Effects last typically quite quickly but only for a short time (up to 4 hours)

Steroids Small molecules, which include a large group with differing actions. Steroid is often used in dermatology to refer to corticosteroids.

Systemic treatment Any treatment which effects the whole body. This includes tablets and injections.

Topical Topical in dermatology means applied to the skin which includes emollients, topical steroids, and other ointments, creams, gels, and foams—not the latest in current affairs!

Vesicle Tiny blister (pocket of fluid) in skin—seen in herpes infection.

Vitamin D Important substance which has many roles in health. Vitamin D is sometimes called the 'sunshine vitamin' as the major source of vitamin d is through a process of sun (UVB radiation) on the skin. Vitamin D can be tricky to get from food naturally as only a few foods have naturally high levels (oily fish). Many foods are now fortified and tablets can be helpful. Skin and oral vitamin D then go through a complicated process through kidneys and liver to become active.

The right level of vitamin D is not known but many people in this country can have low levels in particular in the winter. We know this can be seen in particular in patients with skin problems—partly because they may not feel comfortable exposing their skin.

Wart Caused by human papilloma virus (HPV) virus which makes rough 'keratotic' bumps on skin.

Index

For the benefit of digital users, indexed terms that span two pages (e.g., 52–53) may, on occasion, appear on only one of those pages.

Boxes are indicated by *b* following the page number

depression 23, 137–38
dermatitis artefacta 120
dermographism 44
diet 13–14, 18, 125–26
discoid eczema 27
dithranol 51
doxycycline 60
drug allergy 43
dry skin 25
  isotretinoin 22
  management 33–34

E
eccrine glands 56, 68–69
eczema
  airborne allergies 31
  allergic contact eczema 27, 32
  allergy tests 29–30
  antibiotic overuse 39
  antiseptics 39
  association with other atopic conditions 29
  atopic eczema (dermatitis) 26, 27–29
  bleach in bathwater 39
  calcineurin inhibitors 35
  causes 28
  common condition 7
  contact eczema 27, 31–32
  discoid eczema 27
  dryness 33–34
  eczema herpeticum 39–40, 101
  emollient use 33–34
  explaining to other people 136b
  flare-ups 32–33
  food allergy 30–31
  genitals 93
  growing out of 29
  infections 37–40
  inflammation 34–36
  irritant avoidance 33–34
  irritant contact eczema 27, 31–32
  itching and scratching 37–40, 38b
  novel treatments 40–41
  seborrheic eczema 27, 39
  steroids 34–35, 35b, 36
  steroid withdrawal syndrome 36b
  symptomatic treatment 40
  types 26–27
education 132
emollients 33–34, 51

exercise 53–54, 126
exposure 141

F
fexofenadine 45
fingernail psoriasis 48–49
flare-ups
  eczema 32–33
  hidradenitis suppurativa 56, 58–59, 60
  psoriasis 48
food
  acne/spots 13–14, 18
  allergies 30–31, 43–44
  balanced diet 125–26
Fordyce spots 92
freckles 83
fungal infections 104–6

G
gender transition 15
genitals/genital skin 90–95
  Crohn's disease 93
  eczema 93
  hair 74, 91
  herpes 101
  infections 95
  lichen planus 94–95
  lichen sclerosus 94
  normal stages of development 90–91
  psoriasis 52, 93
  skin conditions affecting 93–95
  variants of normal 91–92
  vitiligo 88
glands 56–58
  apocrine glands 55, 56–58
  eccrine glands 56, 68–69
  sebaceous glands 56
goosebumps 26
gratefulness 143
guttate psoriasis 48

H
habit reversal training 139
habits 113
hair
  excess (hirsutism) 75
  follicles 11–12, 73–74
  genital 74, 91
  loss *see* alopecia